# The Miraculous World
## of Your Unborn Baby

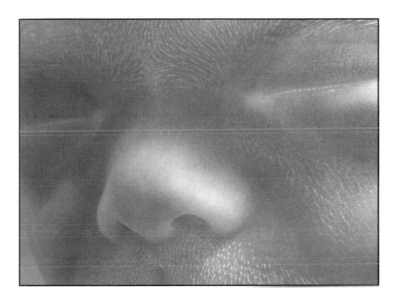

# The Miraculous World *of Your* Unborn Baby

## A Week-by-Week Guide to Your Pregnancy

NIKKI BRADFORD

*Introduction by Dr. David B. Chamberlain*
*President of the International Association for Pre- and Perinatal Psychology and Health*

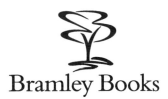

Bramley Books

## SPECIAL THANKS TO:

My editor, Alison Moore, at Book Creation Services (without whom this book would never have seen the light of day). For their help and encouragement, Dr. Ludwig Janus in Heidelberg, President of the International Society for Prenatal and Perinatal Psychology and Medicine (ISPPPM); Peter Fedor-Freyburg, Professor of Obstetrics in Stockholm, Editor-in-Chief of the *International Journal of Prenatal and Perinatal Psychology and Medicine* and Life (Hon.) President of the ISPPPM.

And finally, a special acknowledgement to Canadian psychiatrist Dr. Thomas Verny, arguably the godfather of prenatal psychology, for the inspiration of his book, *The Secret Life of the Unborn Child*.

4981 The Miraculous World of Your Unborn Baby
Produced by CLB International,
a division of Quadrillion Publishing Limited.,
Godalming, Surrey, GU7 1XW, United Kingdom.

This edition published in 1998 by Bramley Books

ISBN 1-85833-966-9

Text commissioned by Book Creation Services Ltd, London
Edited, designed, and typeset by Book Creation Services

For Quadrillion:
Director of Editorial: Will Steeds

Illustrations by Liz Pyle, Sally Holmes, Bob Abrahams, and Sue Rose
Picture research by Jan Croot
Index by Marie Lorimer

Design by Casebourne Rose Design Associates, Brighton
Printed in Spain

# Contents

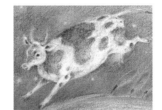

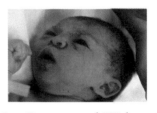

# Introduction

by David B. Chamberlain, Ph.D.

This book is packed with the latest scientific information couples want to know about pregnancy and the developing baby, including much that is new and surprising about babies themselves. These photographs of life in the womb, which have amazed people throughout the world, have the power to end generations of speculation and argument about pregnancy, birth and babies.

Now that we can see with our own eyes what babies are doing in their hitherto private world, we should be ready to assign the highest priority to the all-important first stage of life—from conception to birth. How little our Western culture has traditionally valued this time is revealed by the fact that we do not count the first nine months in calculating a person's age. Pregnancy has been described as a "waiting period", a time "expecting" a future event, a calm before the storm of parenthood. Gestation seemed an automatic physiological process, a grace period during which the baby grew in a protective cocoon safe from (and oblivious to) the perils of the world

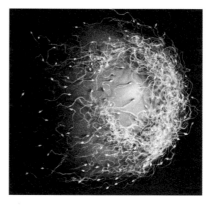

Most of the world has yet to wake up to the meaning of the painstaking, piecemeal discoveries of scientific investigation about the first nine months of life—discoveries that have rendered obsolete most of what we thought we knew only 25 years ago. When seen as a whole, the findings are revolutionary, forcing us to formulate new ideas about both unborn and newborn babies.

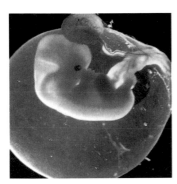

outside. In reality, parenting is in full force even before conception, when the impact of decisions and lifestyle are already having an effect upon the formation of the future child.

In only a brief span of years, the old view that babies were virtually deaf, dumb and blind has been replaced with the view that sensory development in the womb is rapid, voluntary motion comes early and prenates are in constant interaction with their parents— shaping the future day by day. Babies as yet unborn are listening and learning.

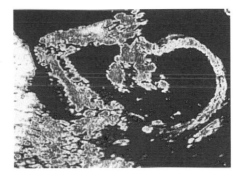

The womb, our first environment, is a very stimulating place, and, whether they realize it or not, parents are major players in constructing each baby's physical body and brain, building each newborn's emotional foundations, and establishing an infant's pattern for relating to others. For good or for ill, this is basic equipment that will serve a person for a lifetime.

*The Miraculous World of Your Unborn Baby* is a reliable guide to current thinking on pregnancy and the development of the unborn baby. When you open this book, whether you are already pregnant or are just contemplating having a baby, be prepared for a captivating new vision of who babies really are and what it means to participate with your baby in the adventure of parenting and childbirth.

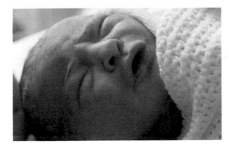

*David B. Chamberlain*

David B. Chamberlain, Ph.D.
President of the International Association
for Pre- and Perinatal Psychology and Health.

# Genetics

## How and why does your baby grow into an infant, a child and finally an adult with his or her own, totally unique character and appearance?

The answer lies in the science of genetics, the study of heredity. Although children's personality traits and intellectual capabilities are a combination of hereditary and environmental influences, every aspect of their physical make-up (whether they are blue-eyed or short, for example) is entirely due to the former, coming from either their mother or father.

These physical characteristics—and there are thousands of them—are all passed on to your baby because each one is controlled by a specific individual information package. These packages are made from deoxyribonucleic acid (DNA) and are called genes. Each is located on a specific site on one of the series of link-sausage-shaped structures called chromosomes, which are con-

tained within the nucleus of every cell in the body. Every chromosome carries many thousands of genes. Each one represents a different potential characteristic for your future baby.

There are 23 pairs of chromosomes in every cell. In each pair, one chromosome comes from the egg ripened and released by you, the mother; the other comes from the

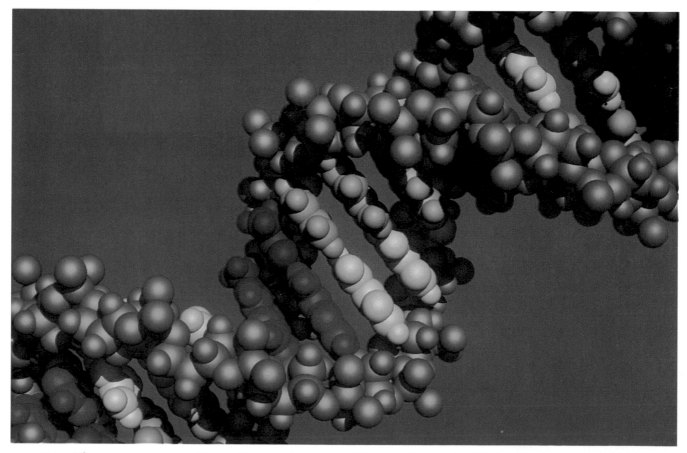

*ABOVE: This computer-generated image illustrates just one small part of the complex DNA molecule, present inside every single living cell. It contains a blueprint for life—and every person's is different.*

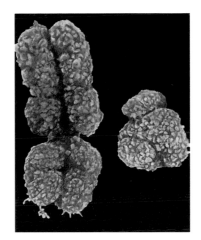

*ABOVE: These are the X and Y sex chromosomes which determine a baby's sex—they are so called because they are (roughly!) X- and Y-shaped.*

*LEFT: Human chromosomes: they carry a person's unique genetic information, and will make exact copies of themselves while the cell is resting between divisions.*

## HOW CHARACTERISTICS ARE INHERITED

This diagram illustrates how a baby inherits traits from the mother and father: in this case it shows whether he or she will have blue or brown eyes. The blue-eyed gene is recessive (weaker) and the brown is dominant (stronger). A brown-eyed mother carrying a recessive blue-eyed gene will only have a blue-eyed baby if she has a brown-eyed partner *also* carrying a recessive blue gene—or a partner who has blue eyes himself.

✖ chromosome carrying blue eye gene

brown-eyed person

✖ chromosome carrying brown eye gene

blue-eyed person

Mother    Father    Mother    Father

Their children    Their children

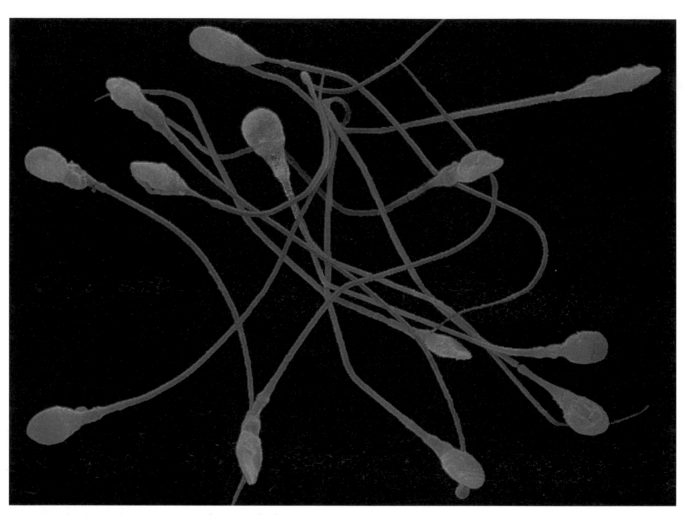

*ABOVE: Sperm swimming strongly, magnified x 1,100. They have been colour-coded to show which ones would help create a girl baby (pink) and which would produce a boy (blue).*

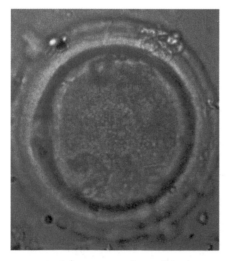

*ABOVE: A human egg (ovum) is shown in the Fallopian tube.*

particular sperm cell, made by the baby's father, which reached and fertilized your egg.

During fertilization, the egg's nucleus, with all your genetic information, merges with the sperm's nucleus, which contains all your partner's. This creates a living mass of genetic material which both initiates and drives forward the complete development of your baby, inside the womb and outside, for the rest of his or her life.

Any genetic error or damage to this vital set of genes may affect your future baby. Genetic problems or malfunctions cause about 60 per cent of early miscarriages.

But if there are so many thousands of possible characteristics babies can have, why don't they exhibit more of them? It is because each particular cell only uses a fraction of the total genetic blueprint available. Some genes are more powerful ("dominant") than others and will take precedence over the weaker ("recessive") ones. Take the example of a girl: if a dominant gene for tallness from the father is mixed in with a recessive gene for smallness from the mother, she will grow up tall.

# WHEN TO SEEK GENETIC COUNSELLING

If you or your partner have a family history of an inherited genetic disorder such as haemophilia, or have had an affected baby before, it is a good idea to see a genetic counsellor, preferably before you begin trying to become pregnant. Your obstetrician or general practitioner can refer you to a genetic counselling unit within a major hospital. Clinical experts and advisers there will help you determine the likelihood of any hereditary problem being passed to your baby, by drawing up a detailed family medical history for you and conducting blood tests, as well as discussing whether or not it may be helpful for you to have one or more of the available antenatal tests, such as chorionic villus sampling (CVS; see p. 55) or amniocentesis (see p. 54), which are used to detect specific genetic disorders.

XX grandparents XY

parents

XY

XX parents XY

XX Normal female
XY Normal male
XX Female carrier
XY Male sufferer

XY children XX

### MUSCULAR DYSTROPHY

This diagram shows the manner in which Duchenne muscular dystrophy, a sex-linked disorder, may be passed on. Looking at the children illustrated in the diagram, it should be noted that the male is a sufferer. The female is free of the gene for the disease, although she had a 50 per cent chance of being a carrier.

### DOWN'S SYNDROME

People sometimes think Down's syndrome runs in families because it is a matter of genetics, but this is not the case. Down's syndrome is actually a chromosome disorder, which becomes more likely as a mother gets older, especially after the age of 35, but it can be detected by an amniocentesis test (see p. 54). It arises when a baby has an extra chromosome 21 (that is, there are three rather than two).

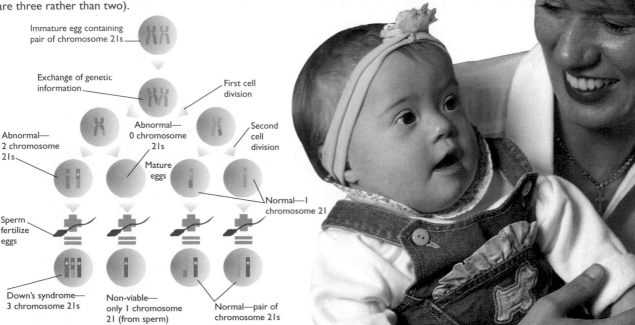

Immature egg containing pair of chromosome 21s

Exchange of genetic information

First cell division

Abnormal— 2 chromosome 21s

Abnormal— 0 chromosome 21s

Second cell division

Mature eggs

Normal—1 chromosome 21

Sperm fertilize eggs

Down's syndrome— 3 chromosome 21s

Non-viable— only 1 chromosome 21 (from sperm)

Normal—pair of chromosome 21s

# Fertilization and Conception

## Fertilization takes place when a sperm penetrates a ripe, waiting egg and their two separate nuclei merge, allowing the chromosomes inside to pair up.

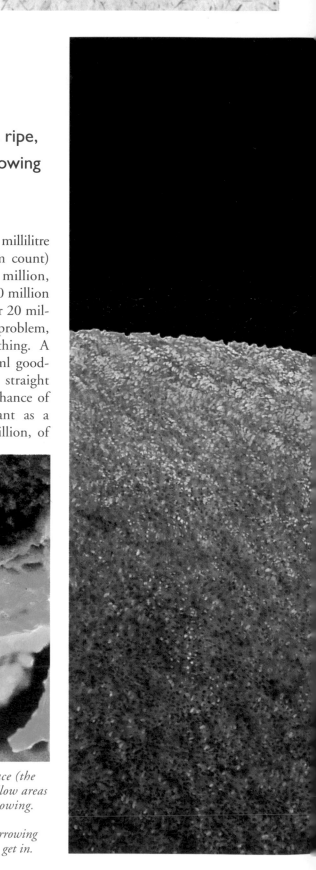

This single new mother cell created when a sperm penetrates an egg is bigger than any other in your body, and is more than 0.1 mm across, about the same thickness as a piece of ordinary-quality typing paper.

However, before you can become properly pregnant, there are four things that need to happen.

First, your male partner must be producing adequate amounts of normal, healthy sperm.

The number of sperm per millilitre (ml) of ejaculate (the sperm count) can be as high as 100 million, although between 60 and 80 million per ml is the average. Under 20 million is thought to suggest a problem, but numbers aren't everything. A man with 10 million per ml good-quality sperm swimming straight and strong has as good a chance of getting his partner pregnant as a man who has 60 to 80 million, of

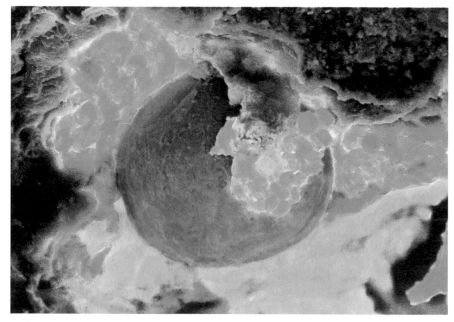

*ABOVE: An egg is released from its ovary, breaking through the thin surface (the germinal epithelium) and into the Fallopian tube. The light green and yellow areas show the cells and liquid which fed and protected it while it was still growing.*

*RIGHT: Touchdown… a sperm has just made it to the egg and can be seen burrowing inside. The outer membrane changes immediately, so no other contender can get in.*

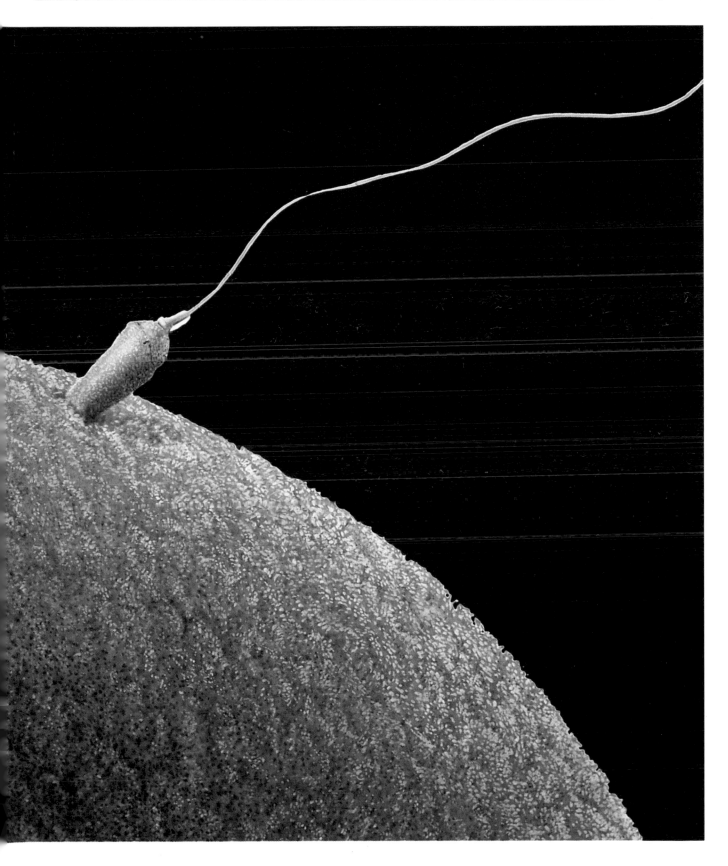

## SPERM—THE FORMULA ONE RACING CARS OF THE BODY

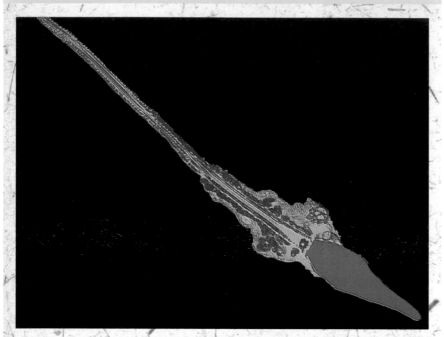

*ABOVE: A single sperm cell—pared down into a bundle of encoded genetic material (the head) and raw energy for movement (the pink areas of the tail are the cellular energy powerhouses, called mitochondria)..*

Sperm are the cellular equivalent of Formula One racing cars. They are lean and honed down, consisting of virtually nothing more than the nucleus (the driver), the mitochondria, or energy-producing mechanisms of the cell (the fuel tank), and a long, whiplash tail (the racing car's engine), which is five times the length of the nucleus. However, the woman's body helps sperm that are doing well: it is thought cervical mucus may contain some nourishment reserves for them, and sometimes the vagina also secretes sperm-friendly alkaline mucus.

*How sperm ripens and matures: from puberty onward, they are produced continuously in the seminiferous tubes (lower left) inside the testes, then stored in the epididymis (above, left).*

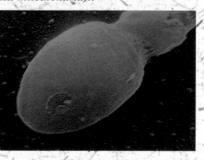

*ABOVE: Head first—a sperm head, magnified x 25,000.*

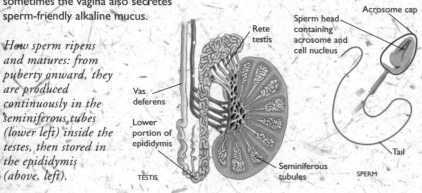

which many are damaged, malformed or swimming too slowly.

These sperm must then be deposited safely near the entrance to your womb (the cervix).

When a man climaxes during sexual intercourse, an average of 250 million sperm—over four times the population of the United Kingdom—is ejaculated into the woman's vagina at a speed of up to 500 cm (200 inches) per second, or 16 km (10 miles) per hour. They then come up against a series of obstacles, including each other. Human fertilization is ruled by the first law of reproduction: that is "survival of the fittest", designed to select only the strongest and best contestant from an enormous number of contenders.

The sperm's first challenge is to withstand the vagina's natural acidity, which does not make for a sperm-friendly environment. The second is to swim through the barrier of mucus which blocks the mouth of the cervix and stops most of the sperm that try to breach it. On a woman's one or two fertile days, this mucus is clear and stretchy, like egg white, and relatively watery, so the sperm can get through it more easily. On non-fertile days each month, it is thick and virtually impenetrable. The third challenge is sheer distance: it is a long way from the cervix to the Fallopian tubes. However, according to Dr. Sammy Lee, a top British consultant embryologist at the Portland Hospital for Women and Children, in London, the sperm that fertilizes the egg can make the journey in as little as 45 minutes, although it can take up to 12 hours. Another senior embryologist, at the fertility clinic in the London Bridge Hospital, likens the

## THE MAIN PHASES OF THE MENSTRUAL CYCLE

The main phases of the menstrual cycle are as follows:

- The egg matures and is released from its ovary.

- Your oestrogen levels rise till mid-cycle, then fall away for a short period as your body makes an increasing amount of progesterone, which in its turn thickens your womb lining so that a 3- or 4-day-old embryo would be able to burrow into it.

- Your mucus becomes clear around ovulation time, then thickens afterwards.

- Your body temperature falls sharply just before you ovulate—then rises again and remains stable.

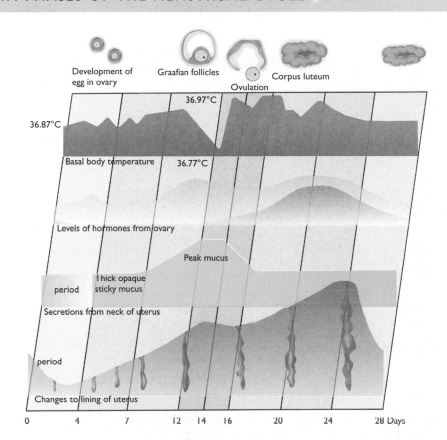

Development of egg in ovary

Graafian follicles

Ovulation

Corpus luteum

36.97°C

36.87°C

Basal body temperature    36.77°C

Levels of hormones from ovary

Peak mucus

Thick opaque sticky mucus

period

Secretions from neck of uterus

period

Changes to lining of uterus

0    4    7    12    14    16    20    24    28 Days

sperm's journey through that mucus barrier to a man having to swim the Atlantic through treacle.

Secondly, you must have produced a ripe, healthy egg from your ovary.

The egg is released into your Fallopian tube and stroked down its length by tiny feelers, like a sea anemone's, called cilia. Your egg can live for about 24 hours, so any sperm must reach it within this time frame. Sperm usually live for 24 to 48 hours, but some have been found alive in the vagina up to 3 days later. This means it is possible to have sexual intercourse two or three days before your ovulation date ("O-day") and still become pregnant. All in all, there is a fertility window of

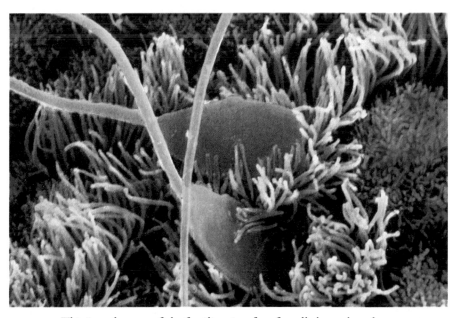

*ABOVE: This is a close-up of the fertilization free-for-all that takes place as sperm fight furiously to be the first to penetrate the waiting egg cell.*

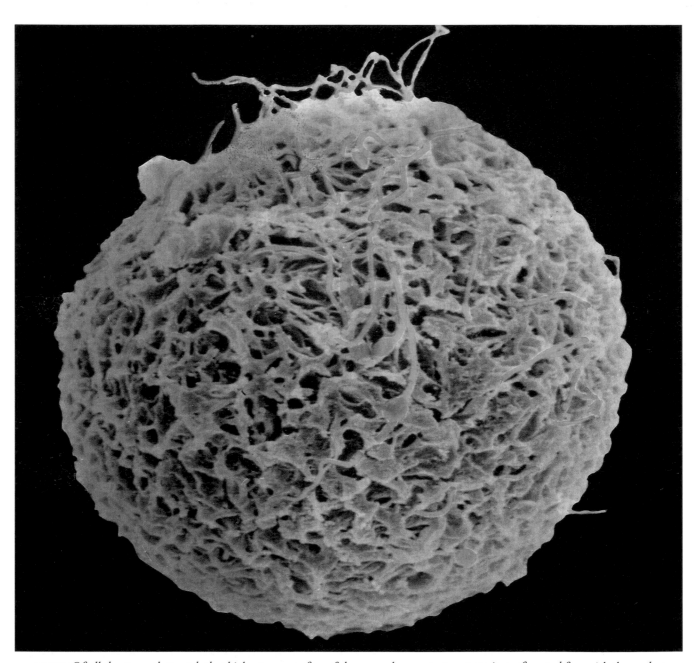

*ABOVE: Of all the sperm that reach the thick, spongy surface of the egg, only one can penetrate its surface and fuse with the nucleus inside. As soon as this happens, the egg membrane changes to form an instant barrier that no other sperm can break through.*

five days—that is, two days before you ovulate, the day of ovulation itself, and two days afterwards. So, contrary to old-fashioned advice, you needn't have sex on O-day or miss your chance for that month—an idea that has long been the source of a considerable amount of stress for couples who were trying to have a baby.

Thirdly, sperm need to be able to find the egg.

According to research in Belgium, sperm are probably drawn to the egg because it releases an "irresistible scent" which they race towards.

Lastly, the winning sperm needs to beat its rivals—down to a few dozen by now—to the egg's surface, and then break in.

Like the bumper on a car, there is a bag of enzymes on the front of the sperm's head called the acrosome. When the sperm hits the egg's sur-

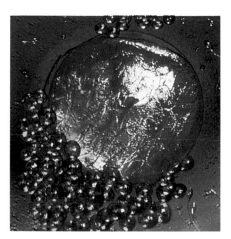

*ABOVE: Only a few hundred sperm have survived the journey through to the egg—as to which one gets in first, it is Darwin's survival of the fittest.*

## OPTIMUM TIMES FOR FERTILIZATION

This chart shows the time when you are most likely to conceive—just after your temperature rises slightly, and when you notice a slippery, stretchy clear mucus discharge. The fertility window is about five days; the optimum time overall is the middle three days.

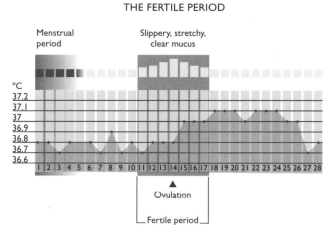

THE FERTILE PERIOD

face, this bursts like an exploding chemical warhead, dissolving part of the egg's protective shell, and creating a gap large enough for the sperm to wriggle through by lashing its tail furiously from side to side. Once the sperm has fused with the egg cell, their genetic material will pair up within about 24 hours, creating 23 pairs of chromosomes from the two single sets of 23. This process, called fertilization, is accompanied by an almost instantaneous change in the egg's outer membrane, so that no other sperm can get inside. On the rare occasion when two sperm do get through at the same moment, the resulting embryo will not last. (Note, though, that twins result from two different sperm combining with two separate eggs, or from a single egg and sperm bundle which splits in half at an early stage.)

Fertilization has now taken place. However, you will not be "properly" pregnant until the embryo, which divides from one cell into a tiny bundle of 64 cells (a morula) in the next 72 hours, reaches your womb and begins to burrow into its lining.

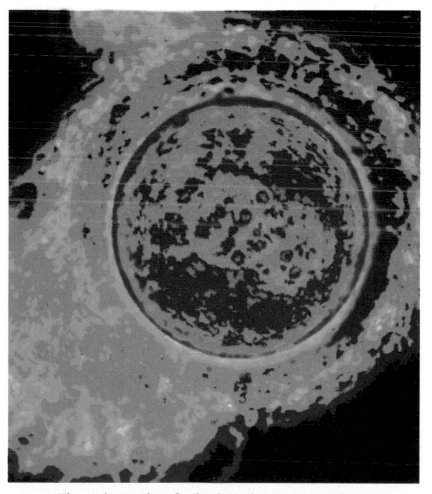

*ABOVE: This egg has just been fertilized. Inside, you can actually see the two cells' nucleii, containing their precious genetic material, merging together.*

# Implantation

Four to five days after conception (fertilization) the cells
have divided to form a blastocyst, a minute hollow ball of about
100 cells, with an outer layer called a trophoblast.

The embryo is still too tiny to be seen by the naked eye. By day seven, it begins sprouting fronds called chorionic villi which will become embedded in any surface on which the blastocyst lands. This is almost always the womb lining—where it is meant to be—but in 1 in every 200 pregnancies the blastocyst burrows into the lining of a Fallopian tube, causing an ectopic pregnancy; this needs to be removed medically or surgically because it can cause life-threatening internal bleeding.

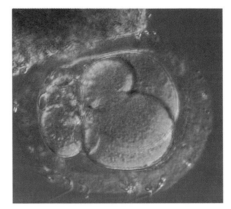

*ABOVE: The very beginning of a human embryo, which will soon become a foetus, then a baby.*

The villi-covered blastocyst normally reaches the womb by the seventh or eighth day after conception. Here it has to anchor itself to the womb wall, burrowing into it by releasing chemicals which eat into a tiny area of the womb lining, usually the upper back wall of the womb. This is implantation, and if it is successful, you are now officially pregnant. The process is not as easy as it sounds, though, and some 40 per cent of conceptions fail at this stage without the mother ever having realized she was pregnant.

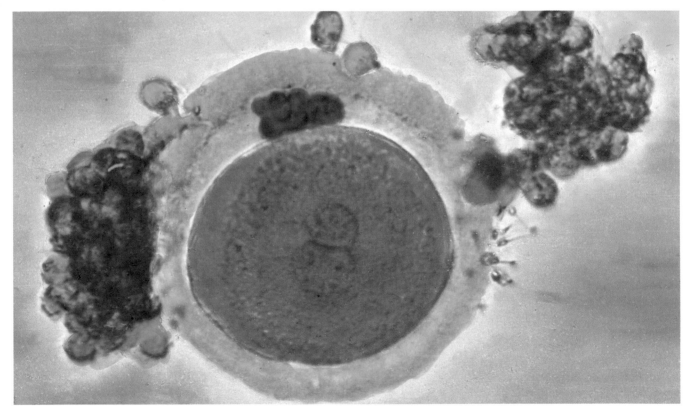

*ABOVE: This shows an egg 24 hours after fertilization—inside, the genetic material from both egg and sperm are coming together.*

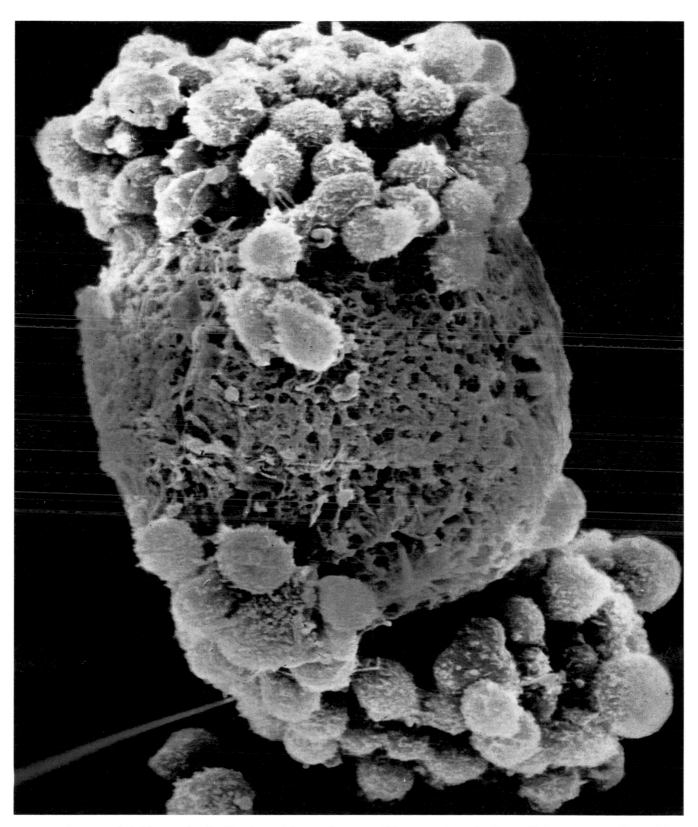

ABOVE: *An egg, only 24 hours after fertilization, with several unsuccessful sperm, coloured yellow, still hanging on to the outside.*

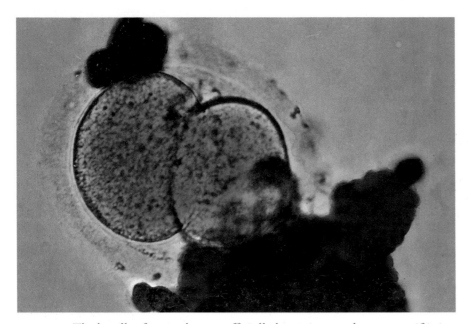

*ABOVE: The bundle of egg and sperm officially becomes an embryo—even if it is only two cells big. This is just 40 hours after fertilization.*

implants, it is sending out chemical messages to you, the mother. These include the hormone human chorionic gonadotrophin (HCG) which pregnancy tests detect in your urine. HCG causes the capsule which originally ripened and released your egg to keep making the sex hormone progesterone. This prevents you from having your period as usual, as that would allow your womb lining to disintegrate and be shed as normal from your body in the form of menstrual blood, resulting in the loss of your pregnancy. During the first three months, the placenta gradually takes over the manufacture of progesterone, which keeps your pregnancy stable and secure.

The good news is that in the remaining 60 per cent of cases the blastocyst does manage to "dig" itself a home in the womb lining. This burrowing process also helps provide the embryo with its first real nourishment, consisting of fats, proteins, sugars and other vital nutrients.

The chorionic villi begin to grow into the blood vessels of the womb lining like a plant's roots seeking water, taking in the oxygen and food the developing embryo needs. Blood flows from your broken capillaries into spaces at the thickening base of the embryo and back out again into your veins. This base also starts growing inward, sending out minute tendrils called microvilli into the tissue of the womb lining and, later on, into the womb itself. These microvilli and the thickening base gradually become your baby's placenta.

The blastocyst has quite an effect on your entire system in other ways because, probably even before it

## FERTILIZATION THROUGH TO IMPLANTATION

Shown here are the stages from when the ovary releases a single ripe egg, to that egg's fertilization, its growth into a tiny bundle of cells, called a zygote, and finally its implantation safely into the soft, rich womb lining.

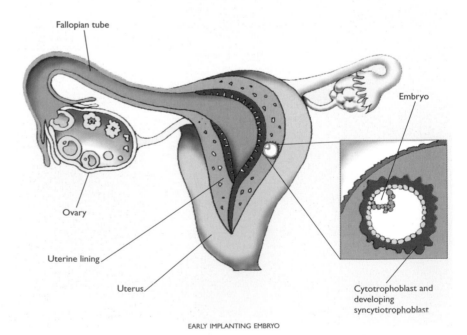

EARLY IMPLANTING EMBRYO

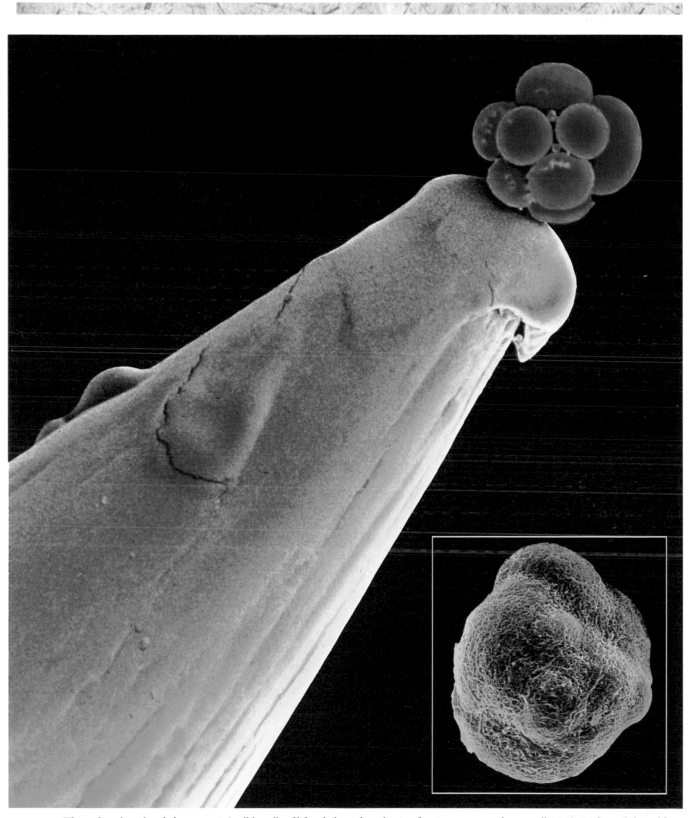

*ABOVE: The embryo has already become a 16-cell bundle of life—balanced on the tip of a pin you can see how small it is (it is about 4 days old).*

*INSET: A human embryo, 3 days old and all of 12 cells big. It now has to implant itself in the womb lining if it is to survive.*

# Natural Gender Selection

### Strictly speaking, the sex of your future baby is determined by the father.

There may be certain ways in which parents can try to increase the likelihood of having a son or daughter (see Your Chance to Choose, p. 24). The way the genetics of sex determination works biologically is outlined below.

A normal female cell has 44 ordinary chromosomes, plus 2 X sex chromosomes (XX). These sex chromosomes are responsible for the development of all specifically female characteristics, such as the breasts, womb and ovaries.

While a normal male cell also contains 44 ordinary chromosomes, plus 2 sex chromosomes, this time only one is an X: the other is a Y, making the male sex chromosome combination XY. It is the Y part

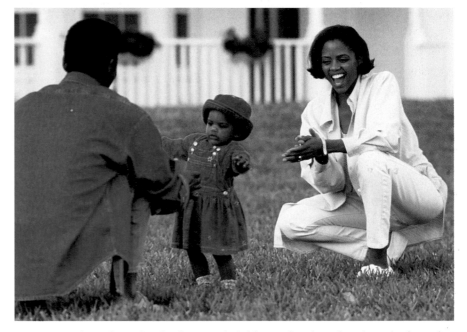

*ABOVE: Baby girls tend to be the second child in a family rather than the first; the "typical" Westernized urban nuclear family ideal of "elder boy, younger girl" is true.*

## STRESS IN MEN—HOW DOES IT AFFECT THE GENDER OF YOUR CHILD?

Men who work in stressful professions—whether it be the psychological stress of big business, or physically more hazardous careers in, say, oil-rig trouble-shooting—father more daughters. No one is quite sure why. Suggested theories have included the possibility that adrenaline, noradrenaline and cortisol hormones produced naturally by the body in response to stress, whether it's sudden and acute or on-going and chronic, may affect the balance of sex hormones in men. This is certainly a factor in general fertility problems for both sexes, and also in certain sorts of period problems in women. So far, though, there's been no proper research conducted into how it affects babies' gender.

*RIGHT: The inheritance of sex—will you have a boy, or a girl? The answer depends on whether the sperm which fertilizes your egg is a "male" (carrying a Y chromosome) or a "female" sperm (carrying an X-chromosome). Eggs are always X-bearing, while sperm may be X or Y. The sex of the child depends on whether an X or Y sperm has fertilized the egg.*

22

which is responsible for the development of all male characteristics, such as the beard and body hair growth, and a deeper voice after puberty.

When sperm cells are made, they are different genetically from any other type of cell in a man's body. This is because instead of containing their usual package of 44 chromosomes plus XY they contain 22 chromosomes plus an X or a Y.

No one is sure of the exact ratio of motile Y-carrying sperm to X-carrying sperm, according to Dr. Sammy Lee, one of Europe's top embryologists. "It may vary from man to man," he says, "because although the ratio should be 50:50, not every sperm in an ejaculate is motile. Non-motile sperm are not useful! Since we are unable to predict whether the loss of motility affects X and Y sperm equally, in some men the effective ratio could be 70:30, for example, while in others it might be the other way around. In yet others it's 50:50, so it's a matter of chance (possibly adjusted by any of the factors listed on p. 25) which one gets to fertilize the waiting ripe egg. If it's a Y-carrying sperm, the resulting baby will be a boy; if it's an X-carrying sperm, it will be a girl."

No one really knows why some families produce a long line of boys, while others have only girls, as statistically the chances of conceiving either a girl or a boy ought to be the same.

ABOVE: *A DNA molecule—DNA contains the inherited code of instructions that control every characteristic of your future baby, including its gender.*

## GENDER FACTS

Listed below are some points to bear in mind about gender.

- Baby girls are rarer in some parts of the world than in others. In Europe and North America, for example, more boy babies than girl babies are born—a ratio of 105:100. In Hong Kong, the figure for boys is 109; in Greece, it is 113; and in Korea and Gambia, 116.

- First-borns are most often boys.

- More boys than girls are born immediately after wars.

- The father's job appears to make a difference. Men in highly stressful careers, such as astronauts, fighter pilots and Australian abalone divers, have more daughters. So, too, do male anaesthetists and men working in bars and breweries. This is possibly due to the chemicals used in modern anaesthesia and the oestrogen-encouraging properties of alcohol.

- The number of boys and girls born varies with the season. In the United States, for example, the peak month for boys is June.

- More daughters are born to older couples. Women treated with the fertility drug Clomiphene are also more likely to have girls.

# Your Chance to Choose

There are many superstitions about how to guarantee a
boy or a girl baby, and couples have tried to influence their
chances ever since the creation of inherited wealth.

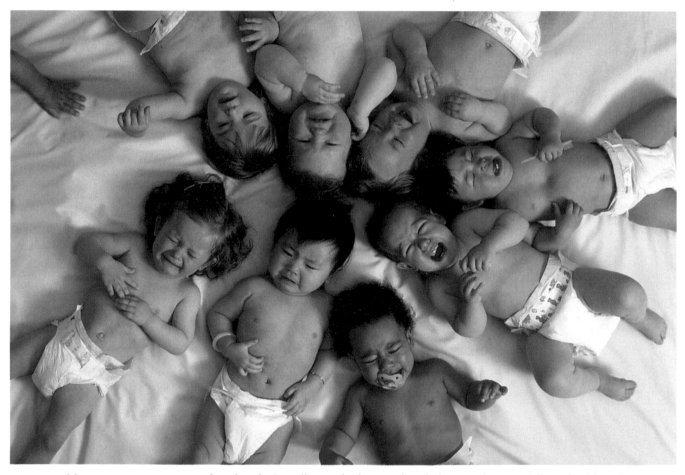

*ABOVE: Most expectant parents say that they don't really mind what sex their baby is, as long as it's born healthy—but some
couples have strong personal preferences and would like to have a say in the matter. Timing and diet may play a part.*

Because the ancient Greeks thought the left-hand testicle provided the seed for girls and the right-hand testicle that for boys, they tried tying off one testicle before making love. Some French noblemen, desperate for a male heir, took this further and had their left testicle surgically removed (without anaesthetic in those days). In the Palau Islands of the Pacific, the wife dresses up in her husband's clothes before making love if she wants to have a boy. Midwives in Austria sometimes still bury the placenta under a nut tree after the birth if requested to do so in the belief that it will guarantee a son next time.

However, since the late 1970s, doctors have been making more of a science of gender preselection. Their research is based on two biological theories, neither of which has been proven, and which have contradictory principles.

First, X- and Y-sperm behave differently. Y-sperm swim faster, but are smaller and do not live as long as the larger, slower but more long-lasting "female" sperm.

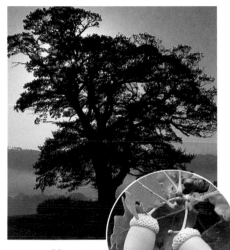

*ABOVE: Nature runs on natural selection, but man can now try to manipulate nature.*

Secondly, male-producing sperm seem to like the acidic environment of the woman's vagina, and survive longer there than the "female" sperm.

### GENDER SELECTION

Both your timing and your diet may affect whether you have a boy or a girl. The first possible method of gender selection is having intercourse at very specific times.

**Based on**: the idea that male sperm swim faster, but that female sperm live longer.

**Action**: first, work out exactly when you ovulate (only 8 per cent of women have the supposedly typical 28-day cycle, ovulating on day 14). You can do this by charting your temperature, but it's easier to check your cervical mucus; if it's clear and stretchy like egg white, you are ovulating. You can also buy an ovulation kit from a pharmacy to test your urine.

This way you can time your unprotected lovemaking to try to guarantee that the desired sperm—"male" or "female"—fertilizes the egg. Making

## HOW IMPORTANT IS SEX SELECTION FOR YOU?

There are pros and cons involved in trying to influence your future child's sex.

| PROS | CONS |
|---|---|
| • Helps to avoid any sex-linked inherited diseases, if there is a family history of such conditions. | • May lead to a greater imbalance between the sexes—probably too many boys. |
| • Provides balance for the typical two-child family. | • Open to potential political and social abuse in totalitarian states. |
| • Less chance of disappointment for parents when they long for either a boy or a girl. | • Failure may lead to great parental disappointment, which could affect the future relationship with the child. |

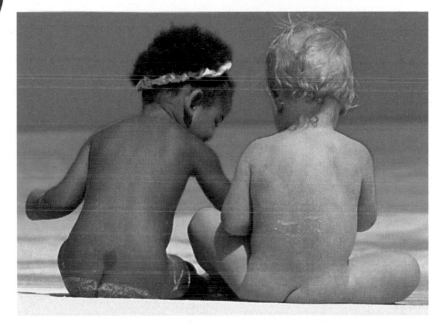

*ABOVE: One boy, one girl—the nuclear family ideal in Western developed countries.*

love on the day of ovulation raises your chances of having a boy, because it is most likely that the faster-moving male sperm will reach the egg first. Making love two days before ovulation day means you have a greater chance of having a girl, as most of the male sperm will have died by the time you ovulate. Even if they do reach your Fallopian tubes ahead of the females, a ripe egg won't have been released yet.

The first doctor to propose this method was Dr. Sophie Kleegman, an infertility specialist practising in New York in the 1950s. She noticed that it made a difference if her patients had artificial insemination treatment on certain days in their menstrual cycle. Her theories have been confirmed by some clinical studies since. There have been other studies (such as those conducted by the researcher William James, of

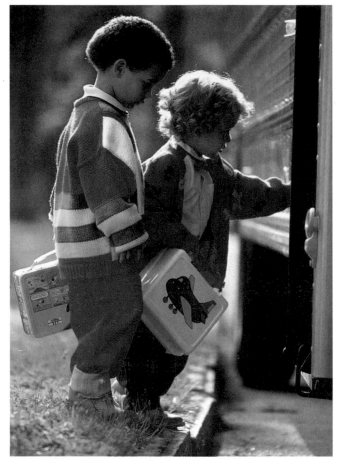

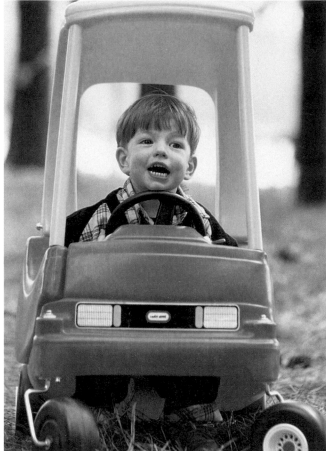

*ABOVE, RIGHT AND BELOW: Whether you have a girl or a boy, babies—and the toddlers, children, adolescents and adults they later become—all have a vibrant, highly individual mix of both assertive, "masculine" and more intuitive, co-operative, gentle, "feminine" characteristics, which make every person an individual. Some of these characteristics are inherited, some develop later as a result of learning, imitation and other environmental factors—and others, such as how the child reacts to stress, are, according to prenatal psychologists, influenced by the different experiences babies have in their mothers' wombs (see p. 59).*

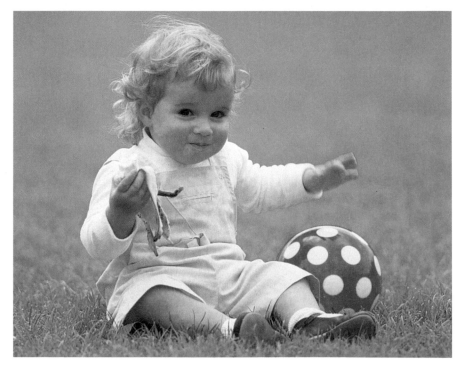

University College, in London), however, which suggest the opposite. Most orthodox medical practitioners still regard sex selection methods with a professionally jaundiced eye.

The second method used to influence your baby's sex, following a specific diet, is still speculative, but the idea has been popular since the mid-1980s, when the appropriately named Dr. François Papa, a French obstetrician at the Port-Royal Maternity Clinic, in Paris, publicized his methods.

**Based on:** the possibility that certain mineral salts affect the likelihood of an X- or Y-bearing sperm fertilizing the waiting egg.

**Action:** if you would like a boy, according to Dr. Papa, eat a diet rich in sodium and potassium; for a girl, eat one that is rich in calcium and magnesium.

## DIETARY ACTION IN SEX SELECTION

Many people believe that sticking to a specific diet or avoiding certain foods can influence the sex of your child.

### FOR A BOY

**Stick to:** plenty of salty foods as well as tea, coffee, alcohol, rice, pasta, meat, fish, milk-free puddings and sauces, cornflakes, white breads, white-flour crispbreads, vegetables (except those in the list for a girl, and raw vegetables, especially cabbage, cauliflower and spinach), all fresh fruits, prunes, raisins, dates, figs, sugar, cooking oil and milk-free margarine.

**Avoid:** milk in any form (for example, yogurts and cheeses), shellfish, pastries, and biscuits containing milk, brown bread, salad vegetables, nuts and chocolate.

### FOR A GIRL

**Stick to:** dairy products such as milk puddings, unsalted cheese, unsalted butter, yogurts and eggs. Make sure you have sweet foods, such as jam, chocolate and honey, once a day. Also eat rice, pasta, semolina, flour, cornflour, unsalted nuts, and plenty of carrots, beans, turnips, onions, leeks, peas, peppers and cucumbers. You should always read labels carefully on packaged foods to make sure that sauces, bread, crispbreads and any other foods are salt-free.

**Avoid:** salt and salted foods.

## WEIGHING UP WHETHER YOUR CHILD'S SEX MATTERS

There are no guarantees with these sex-selection methods. At best they may raise the likelihood of having the baby of the sex you want from the natural 50 per cent to around 80 per cent (although some doctors are claiming success rates of nearly 90 per cent). The most recent development is the separation of "male" and "female" sperm by some sex selection services to use for artificial insemination. However, the medical ethics aspects are still the subject of heated debate, unless the reason is to avoid the strong likelihood of sex-linked inherited disorders, such as haemophilia.

Before you try these methods, ask yourself and your partner these two questions:

- If you already have a son or daughter, would you still like to have another baby in the family, of whatever gender?

- If your new baby did not turn out to be the sex you were hoping for, how would you feel?

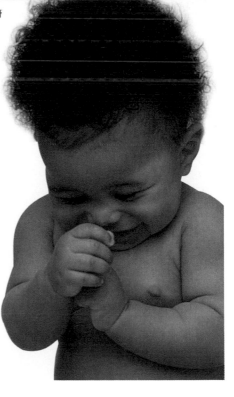
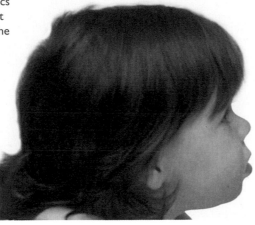

## DAYS 5–17

### EARLY DAYS

- Around the start of this period the embryo is a disc of cells; with so much information stored on it, it is nicknamed the "baby on a compact disc".

- Although only the size of a pinhead by day 11, the embryo already has a yolk sac to supply it with nourishment.

Around day 17 or 18 is a red-letter day for the embryo, and may come just as you are beginning vaguely to wonder why your period is a day or so late. At this time, the flat disc of cells folds into the basic shape your baby will be building on and adding to until birth.

Trophoblast invading the endometrium (implanting)

Trophoblast

There is no other time in a person's life when he or she changes as rapidly or to such an extent as during this time. Professor Lewis Wolpert, the famous British biologist, describes the primitive disc folding as "the most important event in every life".

# The Development of Your Baby in the Womb

This part of the book looks at the beginning of your baby from the embryo stage (up to about day 48, or the 7th week) to the foetal stage, which lasts through to birth.

Your baby's body and all of the biological systems within it—respiratory, circulatory, skeletal, brain, kidneys and liver—are formed in the first six weeks. These are the most vital days of your baby's entire life, and the period in which rapid changes occur.

The embryo, which will become a foetus and then a baby, undergoes more profound changes in the first few weeks than at any other time in his or her existence.

On day 11, the embryo is just a round, flattish, two-layered disc of cells, but with so much information for future developments it's nicknamed the "baby on a compact disc"—albeit one the size of a pinhead. Under a powerful microscope it is possible to see this disc has already formed a yolk sac, which will provide the embryo with next week's food, but that is all. Therefore, it is the embryo's top priority to establish another fuel line to last until birth. Remember the tiny seeking fronds which grew from the blastocyst as it embedded itself unshakeably into the mother's womb? These start multiply-

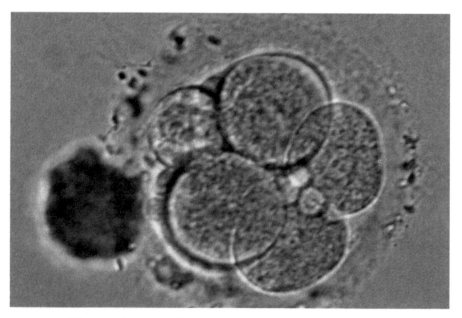

*ABOVE: This tiny human embryo, three to four days old, has been produced in laboratory conditions for IVF fertility treatment. Each cell you can see is called a blastosphere, and could develop into a separate embryo in its own right.*

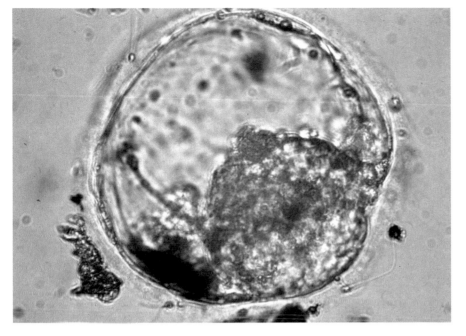

ABOVE: *Five days after fertilization, the embryo has formed into a hollow ball of cells called a blastocyst. It is the circle of cells in the middle of the blastocyst which actually develops into your future baby.*

ing fast now, branching out into an increasingly complex tangle of what are known as villi. The villi link up with the minor blood capillaries in your womb, forming a mass which will, by about the 14-week mark, develop into your baby's total life support system—the placenta.

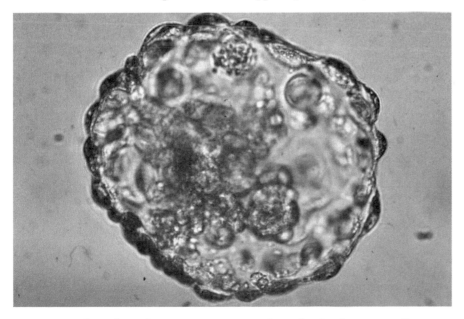

ABOVE: *The embryo shown, just six to seven days after fertilization, will soon implant itself in the womb—at which point the woman is officially pregnant. Implantation is successful in around 40 per cent of cases.*

By day 14 or so, the embryonic disc creates a third layer of tissue within its mass, and every part of your future baby's body will then develop from this triple-layered embryonic disc. Broadly speaking, the first layer will turn into the skin, eyes, ears, nervous system and mammary (breast) glands; the second is designed to be the tonsils, thyroid, intestines, respiratory system, liver, bladder and pancreas; and the third layer is where the bones, muscles, connective tissue, circulatory system and urinary and sex organs develop.

By day 17, the embryo is enclosed in what looks like a tiny bubble called the amniotic sac. The embryo is now also attached to the yolk sac, which, in fact, does not contain yellow yolk as we think of it—the runny yellow part of a soft-boiled egg—but, nevertheless, provides the first vital nutrition in the form of sugars and mineral salts. At this time, the embryo is greyish, jelly-like and translucent without any blood or colouring, like a microscopic caterpillar larva. Also like a larva, it does not give any clue to the astounding transformation about to take place. Caterpillars become brilliant butterflies, and your microscopic blob of living jelly will turn into a human baby with tiny fingers, toes, hair and eyelashes. During the next month you can see how every human embryo fast-forwards through man's links with our animal ancestors, stretching back hundreds of millions of years, as it briefly resembles the embryo of a fish with gills, an amphibian and finally a prototype primate. These evolutionary flashes are fleeting, but unmistakeable.

## DAYS 18–26

### A TIME OF FURIOUS ACTIVITY

- The embryo's future neurological system is a hollow tube containing an estimated 125,000 cells.

- By day 22 the embryo's tiny heart will have started its first contractions, albeit somewhat erratically.

The embryo is now a small C-shaped creature which has a back, a front, a head and a tail end, as well as two of the critical channels which will one day supply it with nerve signals and the ability to process food and to breathe.

Cytotrophoblast

Implanted embryo

Syncytiotrophoblast

Amnion

By day 26 or so, there are signs of relentless activity in the embryo. The optic vessels and eye lenses form, the brain begins to curve forward and limb buds appear, as do the early masses (the primordia) of the liver, pancreas, lungs and heart.

The fourth week of life can be called "brain week", as it is when the three main parts of the brain—the forebrain, the midbrain and the hindbrain—form.

# A Crucial Time in Your Baby's Development

The beginning of the development of your baby's body starts with a small dimple that appears at one edge of the disc of living jelly, which then lengthens into a crack. Cells start pouring towards each other all along the disc's surface, running down into the crack like gravy. They flow into the space between the two layers, plump it out, and later contribute to all of the internal tissues—teeth, bones, muscles, tooth pulp and tendons. During the next three days, half the disc slips down into this groove. The crack then closes up again.

On day 22 or so, the top sheet of cells joins halfway down the groove and the two sides weld themselves together. The resulting hollow tube contains about 125,000 cells—

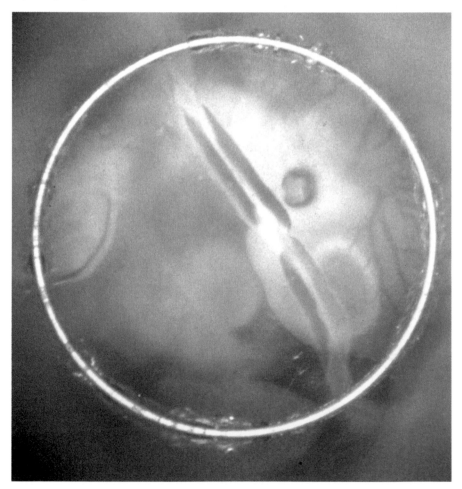

*ABOVE: A living human embryo 26 days old caught on endoscopic camera. Already you can see clearly the future baby's eye (the dark spot) and the developing stomach and heart (middle left).*

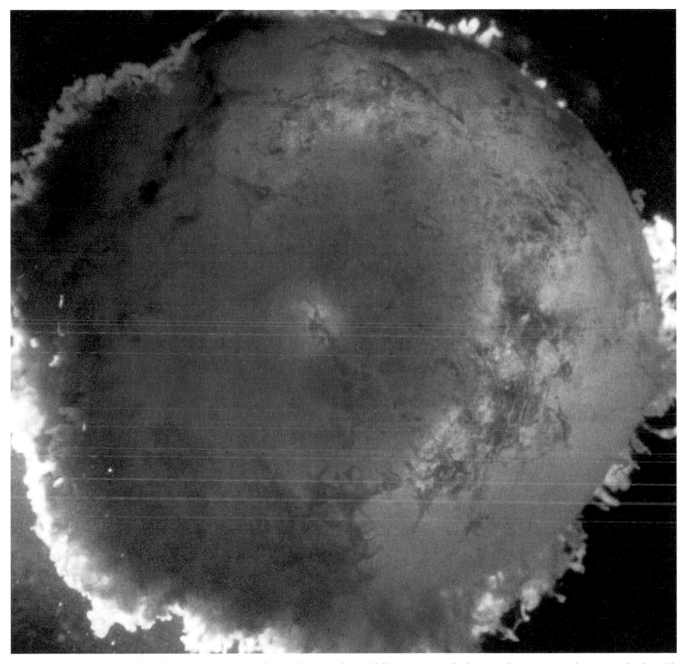

*ABOVE: A four-week-old embryo (you can see the outline in the middle) snug inside layers of protective chorion, which will become the placenta in a few short weeks. The amnion membranes, which grow to form the amniotic sac, are also visible.*

roughly twice the capacity of Wembley Stadium. This tube develops into the spinal cord, brain and network of nerves in the body, and consists of 100 billion cells (about 20 times the population of our planet) when the baby is born.

Very occasionally, the ends of the tube may not close properly, resulting in a birth defect called spina bifida. (Taking folic acid for at least six months before you try to become pregnant reduces the risk.) As this neural tube closes, the edges of the

embryonic disc grow together and downward, nipping off part of the yolk sac—which will be forming red blood cells until the spleen takes over—and creating another tube destined to grow into the baby's throat, digestive system and lungs.

## DAYS 27–38

### RAPID GROWTH

• The embryo at the start of this period is less than 0.5 cm (¹/4 inch) from top to tail.

• The heart is now dividing into chambers and will be starting to develop a more regular rhythm.

Your embryo is growing fast now, at around 1 mm a day. This may not sound like much, but it is actually shooting up overnight by a third, later a quarter, of its body size. By day 36, the head, while still only the size of a small pea, is noticeably larger than the body.

Body stalk

Chorionic villi forming

Developing embryo

Amnion

The facial features are finally developing: the nostrils have slight overhanging borders; the eyes have a dark, tar-coloured tinge from the earliest retinal pigment; and small mounds (called auricular hillocks), have appeared on both sides of the head where the ears will form.

# Intense Activity Continues—Both Inside and Out

Around day 27, the embryo is a shrimp-shaped little being, slightly less than 0.5 cm (¹/4 inch) long from the basic head to the rudimentary tail, and visible for the first time to the naked eye. Its arm buds elongate and then divide into distinct segments, which will turn into your baby's hands, arms and shoulders. By day 34, the outlines of what will become the fingers (embryologists call them digital rays) emerge. The leg buds elongate, too, into distinct thigh, leg and foot areas. Between day 28 and day 35, a more mature and rhythmic heartbeat replaces the early form, and the heart has by now divided into two internal

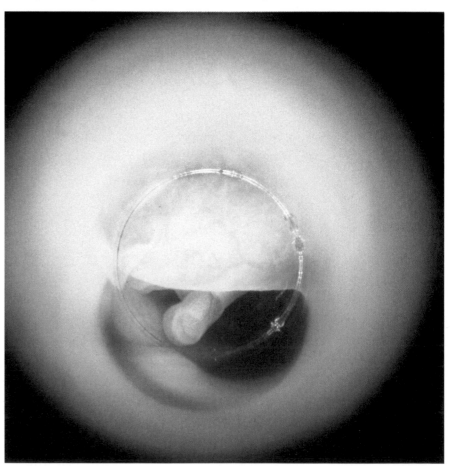

*ABOVE: A five-week-old embryo in the womb—you can see already how its small thumb has developed. Again the shot was taken with an endoscopic camera, which is made from a series of lenses and a fibre-optic light source.*

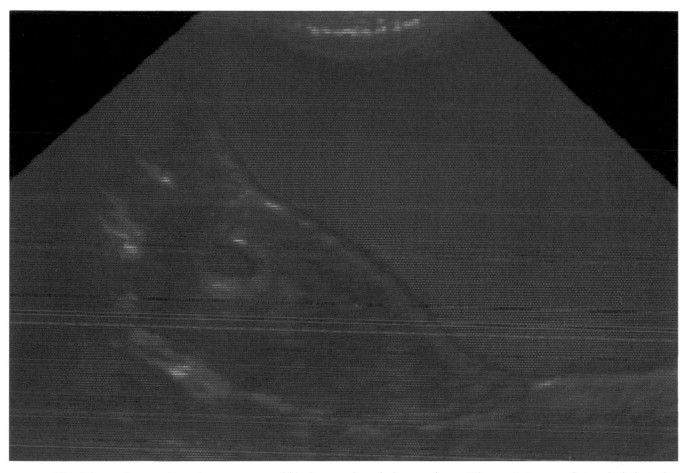

*ABOVE: This is how a four- to six-week pregnancy would look on a coloured ultrasound scan. The amniotic sac enclosing the baby is the small blue oval (centre, left) and the solid blue blob is the embryo's (full) bladder; the mother's cervix is towards the bottom right.*

chambers (eventually there will be four of these).

There is plenty happening around the intestinal area, too, as the embryo develops an appendix—again, harking back to a part of the body our vegetarian animal ancestors needed, but which modern human beings no longer use (it was of more use 10,000 years ago)—and the umbilical cord, which is the embryo's lifeline. The latter is also a chief comforter and plaything until the birth.

By day 38, eyelids have begun to form protectively over the eyes, which will now remain closed for some time. The embryo has elbows

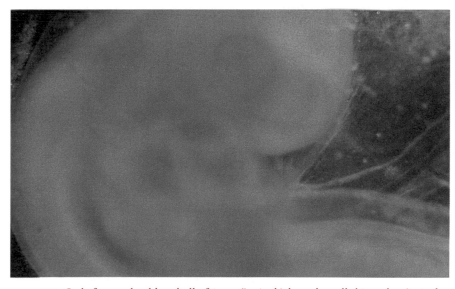

*ABOVE: Only five weeks old and all of 1 cm (1/3 inch) long, but all this embryo's vital organs are developing, including the heart, lungs, liver, pancreas, thyroid and kidneys.*

and finger areas, etched where the knuckles will soon appear. At only 5$^{1}/_{2}$ weeks, the tiny heart would be visible if you underwent a transvaginal ultrasound scan in the hospital. (This is occasionally done if there is some doubt about whether you are definitely pregnant or not, or if an early miscarriage is suspected.) You would be able to see a small dark mass—your future baby—with a tiny pinprick of white light strobing confidently, but erratically, on and off in its very centre.

The placenta, also, will now be growing considerably. The trophoblast layer has sprouted hundreds of tiny villi, making it look like a furry ball. These cells have already been releasing significant amounts of the pregnancy hormone human chorionic gonadotrophin (HCG) into your bloodstream, and from now on its production increases rapidly. It is this HCG hormone that is detected in your urine when you use a pregnancy-testing kit.

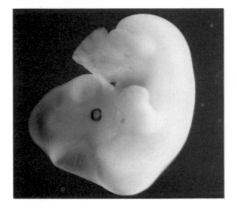

*ABOVE: Four weeks old, but already you can see the limb buds (middle and middle right) and eyes.*

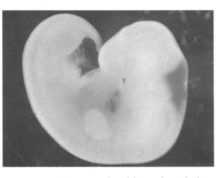

*ABOVE: Five weeks old, and curled into a C-shape because its back is growing faster than its front.*

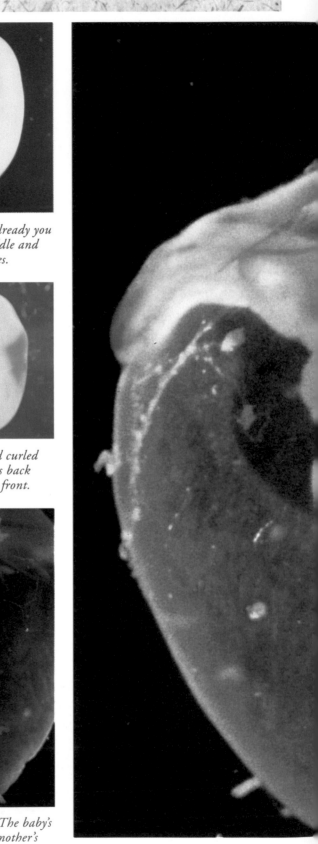

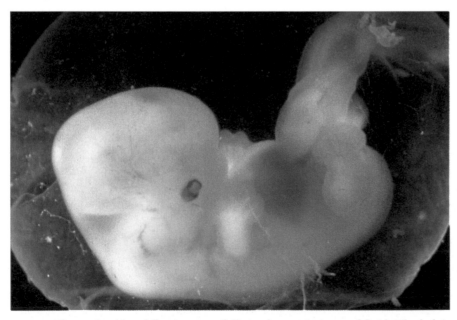

*ABOVE: Six weeks old and floating peacefully in the amniotic sac of fluid. The baby's lifeline—two arteries and one vein—are connecting him or her to the mother's circulation to bring nourishment and oxygen in, and take waste products out.*

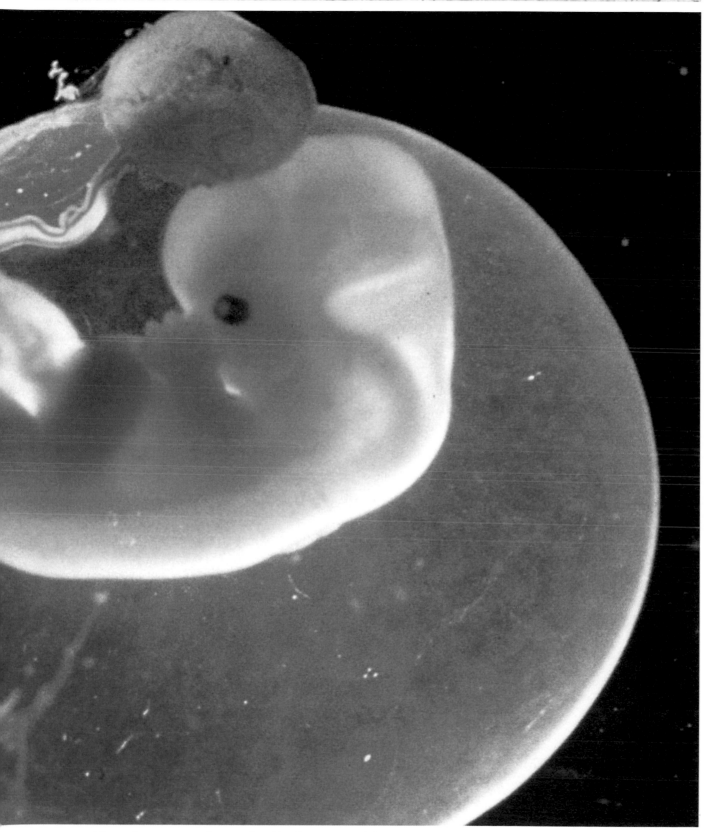

ABOVE: *The embryo at around six weeks old. The remains of the yolk sac are clearly visible above the unborn baby's head.*

## DAYS 39–48

### THE FIRST MOVEMENTS

- Using very sensitive ultrasound equipment, it would now be possible for doctors to see the embryo's first slight movements.

- It is still only three or four weeks since you first missed your period.

It is during the next 10 to 14 days that the embryo really changes its appearance. It transforms itself from looking like a half-human, half-amphibian, delicate little creature to something that is distinctly human in appearance.

Chorion    Embryo

Umbilical cord

During days 38 to 40 the body is elongating and straightening out, with the arms and legs extending forward. The arms become longer, bend at the elbows and curve around slightly over the heart as if in prayer. Two days later, these hands are able to flex at the wrist, while the fingers are longer and the tips slightly rounded and swollen where the sensitive touchpads are forming.

# A Tiny Creature, but Everything's Here

On day 38 or 39, the embryo settles snugly inside a sac of amniotic fluid, and lives there until birth. The warm fluid is 98 to 99 per cent water and keeps the embryo at a constant comfortable temperature. It also acts as a shock absorber and as a cushion against any external pressure.

The embryo's first movements, which can be seen using very sensitive ultrasound equipment, are not complex or coordinated, but the first twitches of a new life are well under way.

By day 42, the embryo's tiny skeleton has been fully formed, not of bone but of its forerunner, malleable gristlelike cartilage. Two days later, on day 44, your future baby has all 5 distinct toes in place, although there is still webbing between them, with a noticeable heel area, and legs which are lengthening daily and have developed knees. The entire embryo has now reached about 2.5 cm (1 inch) in length.

If you could look carefully at the developing face you would see that the eyes, which began forming on both the left and right sides of the head (the same position as a bird's), have moved around to the middle on each side of the top of the embryo's nose. You would also notice that the embryo is able to

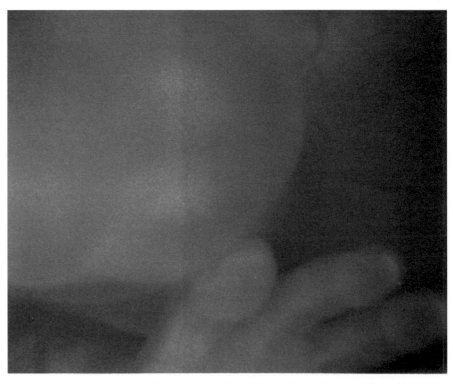

ABOVE: *An embryo's tiny hand is clearly visible, alongside part of the head, in this picture, taken using a fibre-optic endoscope, a sophisticated micro-camera.*

hold his or her head up straighter, and a stout small neck has appeared, whereas only three days ago the head adjoined the body with nothing in between to mark them as separate.

Internally, the embryo's early digestive system is also now in place, as are the kidneys, liver, heart and spleen. The yolk sac, which has been absorbed and contributes to the formation of the intestine, is no longer needed for nutrition, as the villi of the placenta are proliferating rapidly and tapping into your own blood supply for the embryo's food and oxygen.

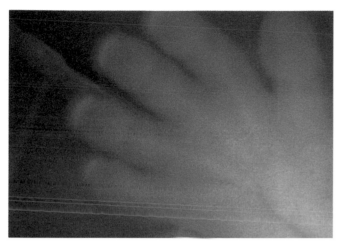

*ABOVE: A close-up of the baby's small hand...*

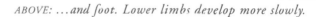

*ABOVE: ...and foot. Lower limbs develop more slowly.*

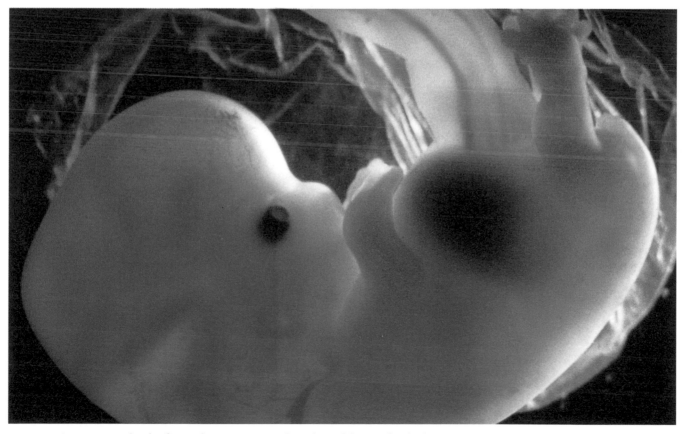

*ABOVE: At seven weeks the foetus has a temporarily enlarged liver (the dark spot) to make red blood cells until the bone marrow develops and takes over the job. The beginnings of a profile are emerging.*

## WEEKS 8–11

### GROWTH IS THE KEY

- Now the embryo is officially called a foetus—the name means "little one".

- At the start of the period, your baby, still only the size of a strawberry—about 4.5 cm (1½ inches)—in length, is about to undergo rapid growth and change.

This period is a major milestone and marks the beginning of a phase of rapid growth, especially between 9 and 20 weeks. It is also a time of further specialization and differentiation of all the organs and tissues formed during the embryonic period (weeks 2 to 7).

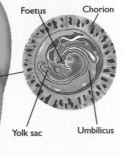

Foetus     Chorion

Yolk sac     Umbilicus

By the end of the first three-month period the foetus will be fully formed: now it is growth which becomes essential, making the foetus far less vulnerable than it was before to the effects of smoking, drugs and alcohol.

# The Embryo Becomes a Foetus

After 8 weeks, the embryo is well-enough developed to become a foetus, the name that is given to all developing babies between the ages of 8 and 40 weeks, until birth.

By the end of 11 weeks the foetus will have grown to just over 8 cm (3 inches). The proportions of the body change rapidly: at week 9, the head is about half the size of the body, yet by week 12 the body length has nearly doubled, and head growth has slowed down.

The muscular system now enters a period of dramatic development, because in weeks 8 and 9 the foetus begins a little arm and leg move-ment, something which you can see clearly on ultrasound. By week 12 they open their mouths in response to touch, begin sucking their fingers, and start swallowing, taking in about 750 ml (1.3 pints) of amniot-ic fluid a day.

Although still made from carti-lage, the skeleton is now developing into a firmer framework. Calcium salts from the blood are deposited to form early bone tissue in the form of a cylinder around the malleable, gristly "bones". From week 10 fin-gernails appear, followed closely by toenails, but they do not yet cover much of the digits' tiny nailbeds.

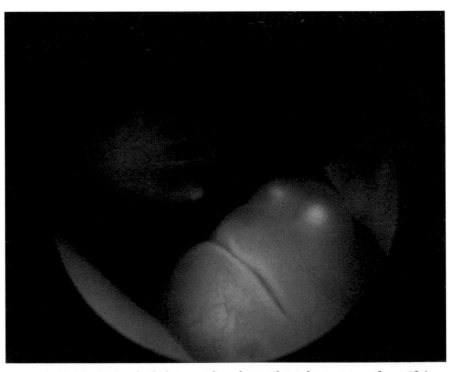

*ABOVE: At ten weeks, the baby's mouth and nostrils are beginning to form. If the two halves of the upper lip and palate do not fuse between six and nine weeks, there is a risk of cleft palate or cleft lip.*

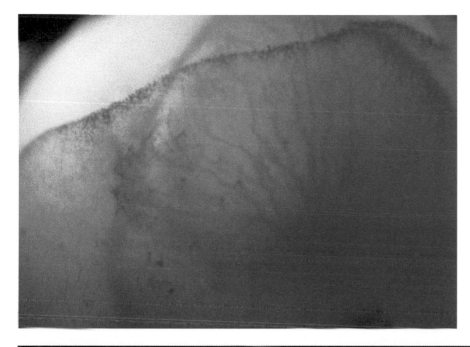

LEFT: *A baby's head at ten weeks, with a temporarily high and bulging forehead, but about to become better proportioned with the overall body size. In this picture the delicate tracery of threadlike blood vessels patterning the skin is clearly visible.*

BELOW: *The baby's eyes have moved down to their proper position on his or her head—and you can say "his" or "her" now as this is also the time when internal sex differentiation starts to take place, though you can see little on the outside. Some of the baby's bones are beginning to become more dense, and to calcify.*

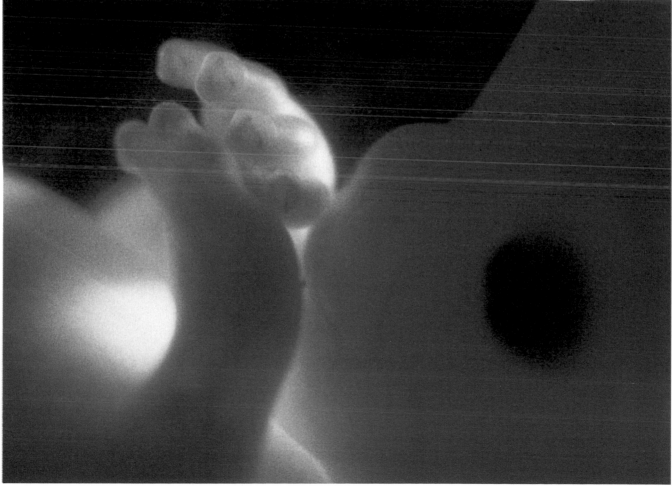

The fingernails reach the end of their fingers only by about week 34; the toenails cover the nailbeds of the toes by about week 36 or 37. However, babies are sometimes born with scratches on their cheeks and foreheads because their small nails have lacerated their skin lightly in the womb. In such cases, the nurse, midwife, mother or paediatrician clips the nails, and perhaps puts cotton "scratch mitts" on the baby's hands for a few days.

The foetus's eyelids meet and fuse together now, staying shut like those of newborn kittens, until week 25. The ears, which began developing on the neck, have moved up to their correct positions on the head.

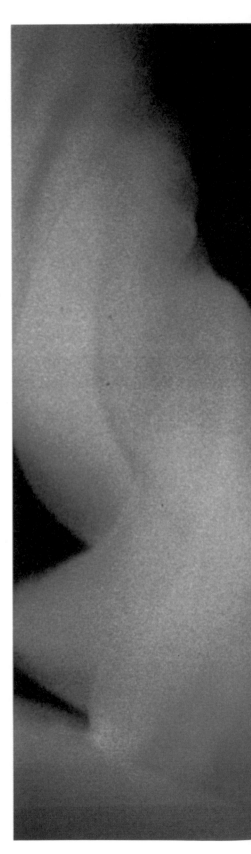

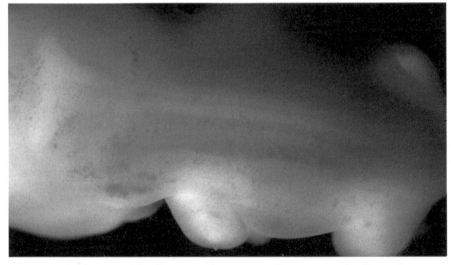

*ABOVE: A back view of the foetus, at about ten weeks. You can clearly see the spine area; the spinal nerves are now growing out from the spinal cord.*

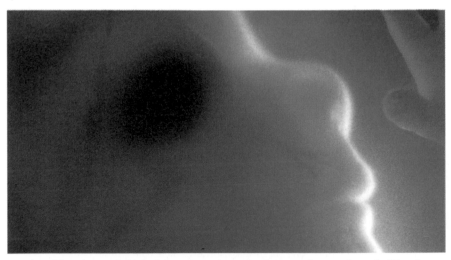

*ABOVE: The retina of the baby's eye at ten weeks, huge and tar-coloured. The change in colouring to blue, brown or green comes at a much later stage.*

*RIGHT: It is around now that babies start making their first uncoordinated leg (and arm) movements: "proper" more rhythmical kicking and movements come later.*

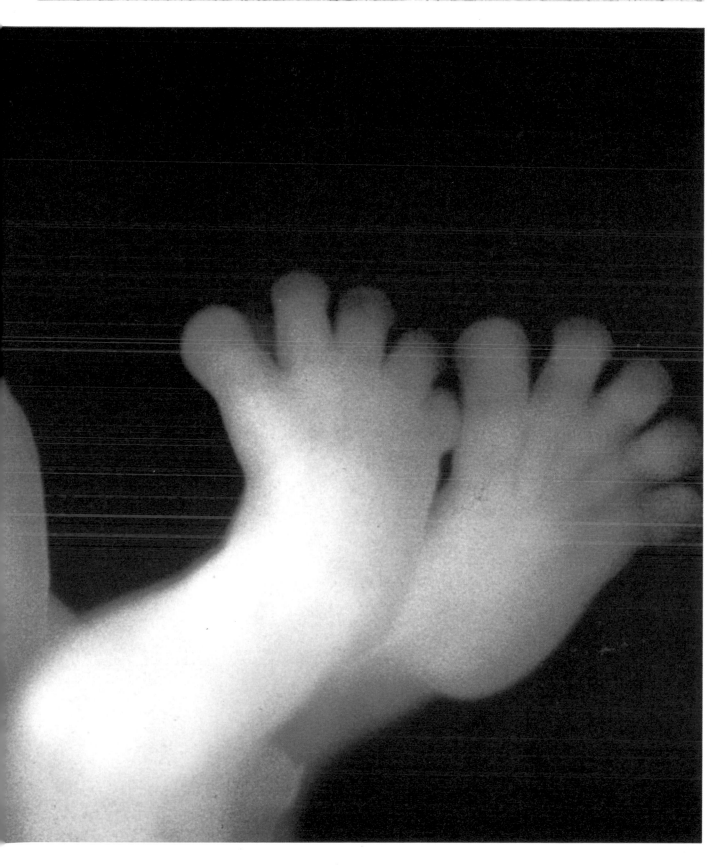

# You at 8 Weeks

Previously the size of a tangerine, your non-pregnant womb has now grown to the size of an apple. Your breasts have become fuller and more sensitive. On your areola, the area of smooth skin around each nipple, you will notice that some small, raised nodules called Montgomery's tubercles have appeared. These are the end points of sebaceous glands which secrete the emollient fluid that keeps your nipples supple for breast-feeding.

Although they are usually a reliable sign of a first pregnancy, they are not such accurate indicators for later pregnancies, however, because they tend not to shrink back completely after childbirth.

Despite all the furious cellular and hormonal activity going on inside you, generated by a tiny being currently the size of a strawberry (see p. 38), there is at the moment little to show for it on the outside except larger breasts, tiredness and, for 80 per cent of women, nausea and/or vomiting—morning sickness. The latter usually starts fading by about week 11 or 12 and is almost always gone by week 16, although a very few women experience it throughout pregnancy and need supportive and careful obstetric monitoring in case they become dehydrated or even malnourished. Caused by the rise in progesterone

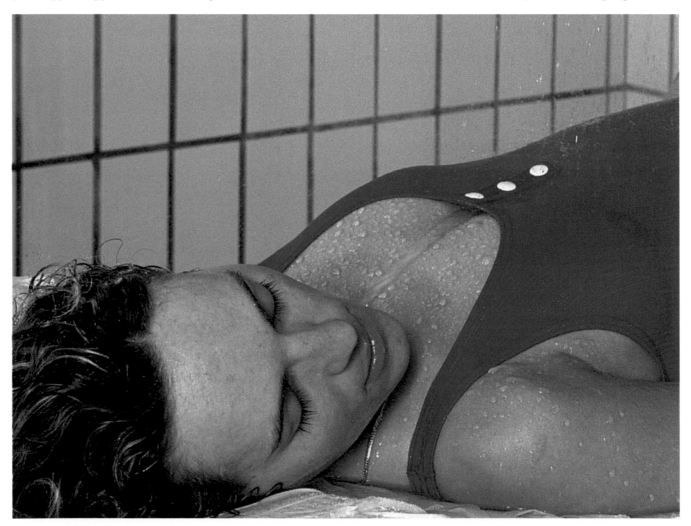

*ABOVE: The very early weeks of pregnancy can make you feel more tired than usual, and most women also feel rather nauseous too. This should pass by weeks 14 to 16, but in the meanwhile try to rest and relax as much as you can.*

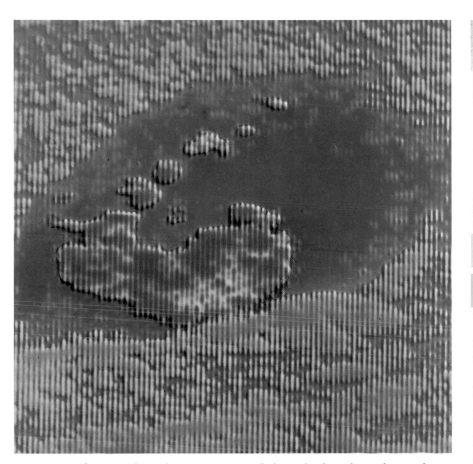

*ABOVE: Even at eight weeks you can see your baby as clearly as this with an early ultrasound scan, although he or she is only around 4.5 cm (1½ inches) long so far.*

### THE FIRST SIGNS OF PREGNANCY

This is the peak time in pregnancy for morning sickness.

Tender breasts

Nausea

Absence of period

#### ANTI-MORNING-SICKNESS MEASURES

- Keep your blood sugar levels up by eating small, regular amounts. Choose snacks or small meals containing complex carbohydrates (bananas, rice, pasta, bread, pizza, baked potatoes), because their sugars are digested slowly and released as a steady supply into your circulatory system.

- Before rising—slowly—nibble a plain or ginger biscuit along with a little sweet tea.

- Take ginger powder (either in capsule form, see below, or as a loose powder, washed down with some water). A 1989 study conducted at the North Devon District Hospital, United Kingdom, also suggested that taking ginger capsules (available from health-food shops) was effective to some extent for 80 per cent of pregnant women with morning sickness.

plus possibly oestrogen and human chorionic gonadotrophin (HCG), the various forms of sickness are thought of as signs of a "good", stable pregnancy because they indicate high levels of the pregnancy-maintaining hormones.

If you find you are feeling very tired during the day, eat frequent, small meals to maintain a constant, stable level of blood sugar, because if this drops you will quickly begin to feel tired, sick and shaky. This condition is called hypoglycaemia. You may currently feel it more acutely because your pregnancy hormones can interfere with the output of insulin, whose job it is to control blood sugar levels.

If you feel the need for real sleep try to find time for a nap. If you have small children, for example, try to arrange even half an hour's regular help at the time you know the exhaustion tends to strike. If you are at work, ask for a designated place to rest briefly. Alternatively, ignore co-workers and put your head on your desk during your lunchbreak. According to research by James Maas, Professor of Psychology at Cornell University, New York, who runs corporate sleep seminars for companies such as IBM and Pepsi, a 20-minute nap between 2 and 3 p.m. is also the optimum time for "power-napping"—any longer and you risk feeling worse afterwards.

## WEEKS 12–16

### THE SEX OF YOUR BABY

- For the first time you will be able to tell on an ultrasound scan whether your baby is a boy or a girl.

- Your baby is now practising breathing movements for the first time.

Around this time your baby's first sexual characteristics develop. The boy's penis is emerging, while a girl's cervix, vagina, womb and ovaries will already have formed.

Umbilical cord Amnion

Placenta Foetus

If the foetus is a girl, she will currently have in her ovaries about 2 million eggs, a number which drops to 1 million by the time she is born. The amount continues to decrease, so by the time a girl is 17 she has roughly 200,000 eggs left, while 20 years later she will only have a few thousand.

# Are You Having a Boy or a Girl?

During this time, or even earlier, you will have the option of an ultrasound scan. On a scan you, your partner and your children will be able to see your baby for the first time and will often be able to tell, perhaps with some guidance from your radiographer or obstetrician, whether your baby is a boy or a girl. Both sexes start off with two internal tubes or ducts called a Müllerian duct and a Wolffian duct. In girls, the Müllerian duct becomes a girl's reproductive tract and the Wolffian duct dissolves away. In boys, the newly formed testes start sending out the male hormone testosterone, turning the Wolffian duct into the reproductive tract and destroying the Müllerian duct.

The first signs of a penis and scrotum may show as early as week 9, but you would need quite a sensitive scan to detect them. By week 12 the picture is clearer, and you can determine whether you are carrying a baby girl or a boy who is a late developer. A girl's cervix, vagina and womb will have formed by now, along with her ovaries.

Between the third and fourth months of pregnancy, your baby's legs grow until they are longer than the arms. In fact, the whole foetus is growing rapidly at this stage: at 13 weeks he or she is nearly 10 cm (4 inches) long, at 14 weeks nearly 11 cm ($4^1/2$ inches) and by 16 weeks, 13.5 cm ($5^1/2$ inches). The skin is rose

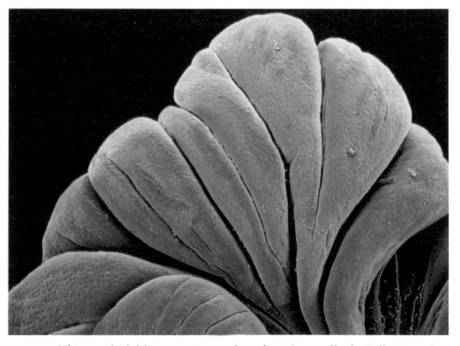

*ABOVE: This may look like an exotic sea plant, but it's actually the Fallopian tube of a 10-week-old female embryo, magnified x 67.*

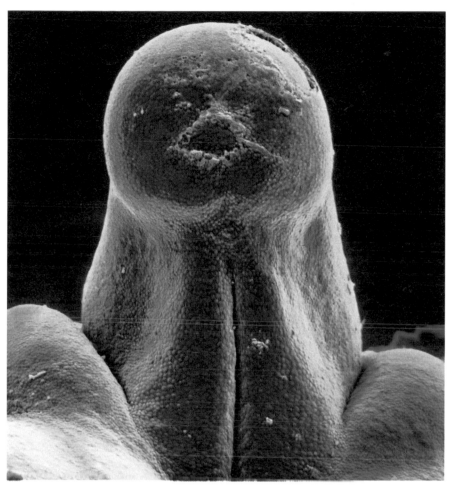

*ABOVE: This may look like a penis, but the opposite is true. Around this stage the male and female genitalia are the same. In fact, this is a picture of what will become the vulva of a girl baby—the round tip will elongate slightly to form a clitoris.*

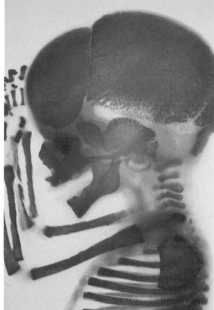

*ABOVE. The baby's tiny skeleton is becoming stronger every day, as it changes from cartilage to bone.*

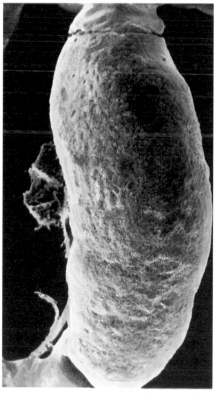

*ABOVE: The ovary (magnified x 90) of an 8-week-old female foetus, who is only 4 cm (1¹/4 inches) long herself.*

red and transparent, so you can easily see the delicate blood vessels forming a complicated and beautiful lacelike fretwork across the head and body.

The skeleton is becoming stronger now, hardening and solidifying as cartilage gradually changes into bone. As more muscle tissue develops progressively, the foetus starts tossing, twisting, kicking and turning, waving his or her arms and moving freely inside the amniotic sac, testing the limits. As growth is now so rapid, this relatively unrestricted space for movement will not last long! He or she can and will also move away from painful or troubling stimuli. For example, foetuses have been observed during amniocentesis (see Antenatal Tests, p. 50) swiping at the encroaching needle, and also trying to get out of its way.

Your baby is now trying out breathing movements, gulping in amniotic fluid and expelling it (see Movement—What do Babies do in There?, p. 47). Much of this will return to its watery environment via the bladder as the foetus practises urinating, but these early spontaneous gasping movements also help train the lungs for breathing air after birth.

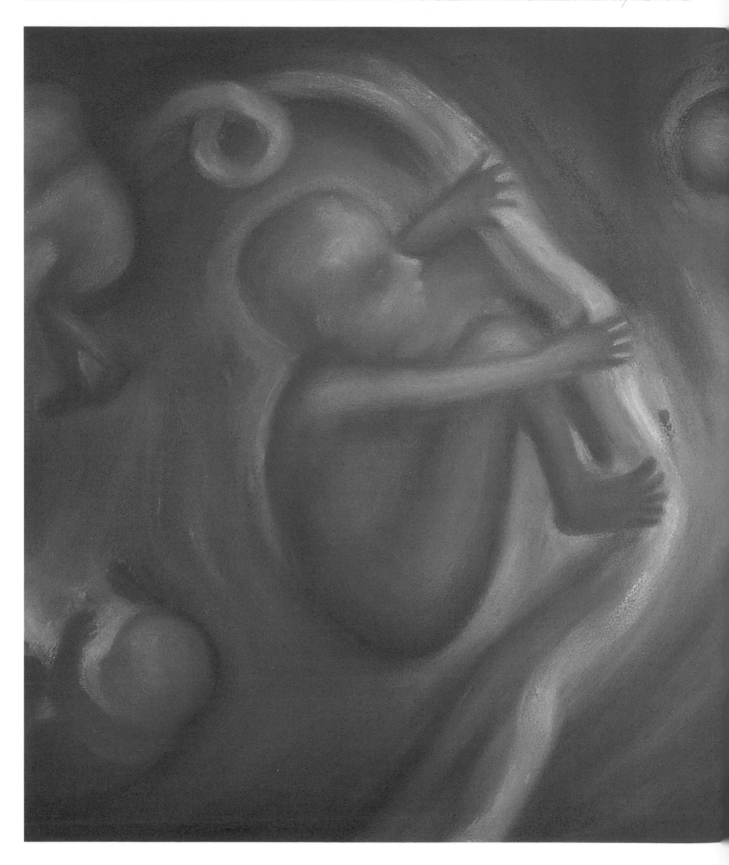

# Movement—What do Babies do in There?

Foetuses spend a lot of time practising the wide range of movements they will need after they are born—a sort of intrauterine body-building programme.

Space permitting, foetuses might be rolling, back flipping, kicking, stretching, yawning, breathing, swallowing, somersaulting, turning their heads, flexing their feet, waving their arms, sucking their thumbs, holding their penises, rolling from side to side, hiccuping and jumping ("startling") at loud noises from outside.

## MOVEMENT IS VITAL

Only if they move a good deal will foetuses be doing enough muscle-work for the joints, bones and muscles to develop properly. But is that all? Are they also experiencing sheer delight in a growing range of movement and uninhibited play? Water, whether it is amniotic fluid surrounding a developing baby, or a pool in which children are free to fool around because of the freedom from gravity its buoyancy offers, is one of the best playgrounds ever created. "Maybe," says Dr. David B. Chamberlain, a top psychologist in San Diego, California, and President of the Association for Pre- and Perinatal Psychology and Health, "it's just fun."

Is all the kicking and rolling working on, and then fine-tuning, the baby's neurological development? Partly that. Also, the more often something is done, the more primed the nervous system is to coordinate the same movements even more smoothly next time. As with an ace tennis serve, practice makes perfect. The same applies for a developing baby. According to research that was conducted in the Netherlands in 1990, if you could look inside your womb to see what your baby was doing at 10 to 12 weeks, you would see that his or her movements are already graceful; French foetal medicine specialist André Boué describes them as "slow, supple and harmonious". They are almost like a restricted underwater tai chi sequence.

## PATTERNS OF ACTION

These bursts of activity may last as long as seven minutes, but it's far more usual for them to continue for only one to two minutes, from the age of about nine weeks. As for foetuses' favourite time to move about, research shows, unfortunately for mothers, that their activity cycle tends to peak around midnight. This is one possible reason why newborn babies seem to be especially wakeful in the middle of the night, until their 24-hour clock settles down to a more sociable pattern corresponding more closely to that of their parents.

In addition to having a favourite time for becoming lively, foetuses also have a favourite place for resting

## WHEN DO BABIES BEGIN TO DO WHAT?

By the three-month mark, foetuses are already able to do most of the things you would expect any newborn baby to do.

| ACTION | WEEKS |
| --- | --- |
| First general movements | 6 weeks |
| Jumping/startling | 8 weeks |
| Hiccuping | 8 to 9 weeks |
| Isolated arm or leg movements | 9 to 10 weeks |
| Chest movements | 10 weeks |
| Stretching | 10 weeks |
| Sucking and swallowing | $10^{1}/_{2}$ to 12 weeks |
| Yawning and jaw movements | 11 to 12 weeks |
| Extending the fingers | 12 weeks |
| Rooting (responding to gentle touch as if searching to suckle on a nipple) | 14 weeks |
| Rhythmical movements of arms and legs | 14 weeks |
| Eye movements | 16 to 18 weeks |
| Making sound vibrations in the womb | 18 weeks |
| Audible crying in the womb (very rare) | 21 weeks |

All the foetal ages given above are based on the date of the mother's last menstrual period, not on the probable date of conception. Some reports give earlier ages for these activities because they calculate the foetal age from the probable date of conception. This gives the impression that foetuses can do things earlier—they can't.

after bursts of possibly tiring movement. Although they may have moved right out of their usual resting position for their regular bouts of gymnastics, they always return to rest back in the lowest part of the amniotic sac.

Unborn babies begin their physical training programmes when young. Sensitive ultrasound tests at the University Hospital of Oostersingel, in the Netherlands, discovered babies begin their first movements at $7^{1}/_{2}$ weeks, while less than 2.5 cm (1 inch) long—about the size of a broad bean. You cannot actually feel them doing

so until the 16- to 20-week mark, but when you first sense their movements, what you will probably notice is a sudden fluttering or tickling, as if there were a butterfly brushing against the inside of your abdomen. Towards the end of pregnancy, the movements will be recognizable as powerful kicks and punches, which, some mothers report, can literally take the breath away.

### YOUR FEELINGS

If you have not felt your baby move for some time and feel worried, eat something sweet and lie down quietly on your left side; you should feel

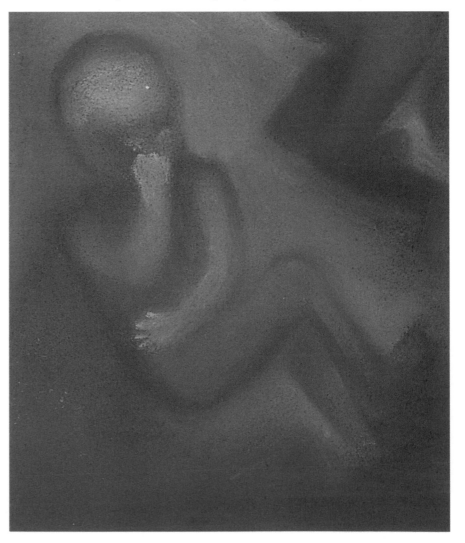

the fluttering or kicking within about 20 minutes as the sugar is absorbed via the placenta into your baby's system. This is because the sugar gives the foetus a hit of energy, which usually encourages a burst of movement. If you don't feel any movement after that, or are generally concerned (perhaps your baby has always been very active at regular intervals and suddenly stops for many hours), immediately contact your obstetrician, GP, the antenatal department of the hospital caring for you during your pregnancy or your midwife. They will not think you are fussing needlessly, but will instead see you straight away, and possibly check your baby on ultrasound to confirm everything is as it should be.

On the whole, unborn babies tend not to stay still for long—though there are reports of them remaining stock-still for up to two hours after a needle has invaded their territory during an amniocentesis test. Mostly, though, they are very lively—research by the University Hospital of Gronigen in the Netherlands in 1985 found that they were never still for more than 13 minutes at a time during the 8- to 19-week stage.

## YOUR BABY'S REPERTOIRE

Your baby will have perfected the full repertoire of these movements by about 15 weeks, and will shift about the most between 13 to 17 weeks, after which he or she will begin to calm down and move less. According to researchers at Erasmus University, in Rotterdam, the gradual slowing down is only partly

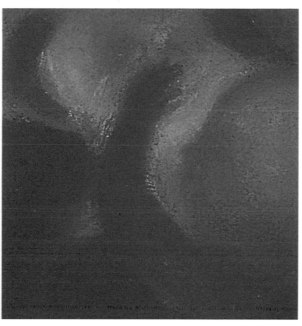

due to your baby getting bigger and increasingly running out of room for manoeuvre. It also occurs because it reflects central nervous system development—different patterns or types of movement serve to strengthen and develop different nerve connections and pathways within the baby's neurological system.

Big movements, such as back flips, rolls and kicks, tend to happen most in the earlier part of pregnancy, whereas lesser activity, such as eye movement, begins at about 16 weeks and increases steadily from then on. So too do any vital mechanisms needed for survival outside, such as breathing movements. These are not breathing as such, which would mean taking amniotic fluid into the foetus's lungs, but practice chest movements, the forerunner to breathing air. Foetuses start making these movements occasionally from about 10 weeks. Activity takes place at a rate of 6 per cent at 19 weeks, rising to about 36 per cent at the end of pregnancy, in preparation for the baby's life outside the womb.

## NOISES IN THE WOMB

Once dismissed as sentimental rubbish, it now seems that, yes, babies do practise making sounds in the womb. Foetuses can be seen on ultrasound using their larynxes not for swallowing or for breathing movements, but for producing sound vibrations from the age of 18 weeks, according to research conducted in 1996 at Hospital Xeral de Vigo, in Pontevedra, in Spain. This discovery gives new support to previous observations that it is possible for a foetus to cry when some air has been introduced into the womb usually as a result of an obstetric intervention rupturing the membranes (amniotic sac). In medical literature, there are 140 documented cases of babies heard crying in the womb, usually caused by obstetric manipulations before birth. It seems that anything which allows some air into the amniotic sac could help in creating the conditions that an unborn baby needs to make sound (without air, sound cannot travel or, indeed, be made). It is possible that an unborn baby could make noises even around 18 weeks. Detailed ultrasound studies made as part of the research showed that "phonetic function", using the unborn child's vocal cords and epiglottis, goes on from week 18. Vibrations from the glottis opening or closing—which may produce sound waves you could hear if they were made in the air rather than in amniotic fluid—are being made from the same time. Audible crying has also been recorded at 21 weeks in some cases of therapeutic pregnancy termination.

# Checking Your Baby's Well-Being in the Womb

"The vast majority of babies are born normal irrespective of the age of their parents," says a spokesperson for the Harris Birthright Research Centre for Foetal Medicine, in London.

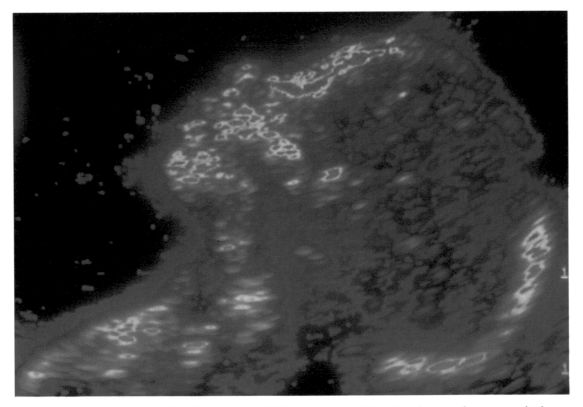

*ABOVE: The face in pure profile of a 22-week-old foetus, seen on a Doppler ultrasound scanner, which uses high-frequency sound waves to check that the child is developing normally.*

Parents often find having antenatal tests and waiting for the outcome stressful, especially if the tests involved an invasive procedure, such as amniocentesis. Yet the results are usually reassuring, and generally confirm for parents that their baby is fine.

However, birth defects, which foetal tests check for, do occur and can be grouped into three categories: physical problems, such as a malformation; an inherited gene defect, such as cystic fibrosis or haemophilia; or chromosomal disorders, such as Down's syndrome.

In the UK, of the 650,000 babies born every year, only about 22,000 will have one of these physical problems, many of which will be minor. Yet, the possibility that there may be something wrong with their (probably healthy) developing baby occurs to most pregnant women forcibly at least once. For others, it is an ever-present worry they cannot get out of their minds. That is where foetal testing comes in.

### ANTENATAL TESTS

For couples without a family history of genetic problems, antenatal tests largely provide peace of mind. For those who do have a history of specific difficulties or who are 35 years old or older (after which point the risk of certain difficulties such as Down's syndrome rises sharply), foetal tests can represent more.

It's a fact that all women, no matter how old or young they are, have a very small risk of having a baby with a physical or mental defect. Using the possibility of a major chromosomal abnormality, such as Down's syndrome, as an example, the figures are: 1 chance in 1,500 if you are 25 years old; 1 in 800 if you are 30; 1 in 350 when you are 35; and 1 in 100 if you are 40—the risks accelerate after your mid-thirties. Down's syndrome babies are always thought to be more common for older mothers, yet the greater proportion are actually born to mothers who are under 35.

This is partly because many affected babies are not detected

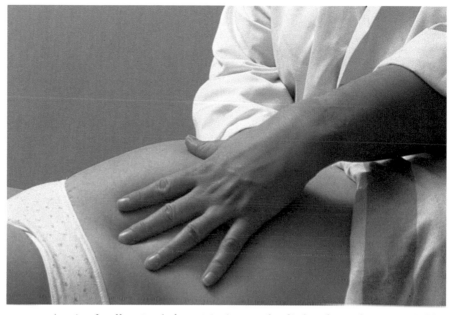

*ABOVE: A pair of well-trained obstetrician's or midwife's hands can be just as skilful when it comes to assessing the size and position of your baby as using sophisticated high-tech scanning equipment.*

while they are in the womb as their mothers are thought to be too young (and their chance of age-related genetic defects considered too small) to warrant an invasive diagnostic test, such as amniocentesis.

Most pregnant women in the United Kingdom are routinely offered screening tests. These involve taking a sample of blood and checking the levels of different proteins, for example, and perhaps culturing and checking the stray foetal cells it also contains. Such simple tests can, at certain research centres, be followed up by detailed ultrasound scans if they indicate the possibility of abnormality, and, if necessary, by more invasive diagnostic tests such as amniocentesis and chorionic villus sampling (CVS, see p. 55), which should provide definitive answers. Screening tests assess the likelihood of your baby having a problem; diagnostic procedures zone in to take a closer, confirming look. Remember, though, that you are not obliged to have any of the tests if you do not wish to.

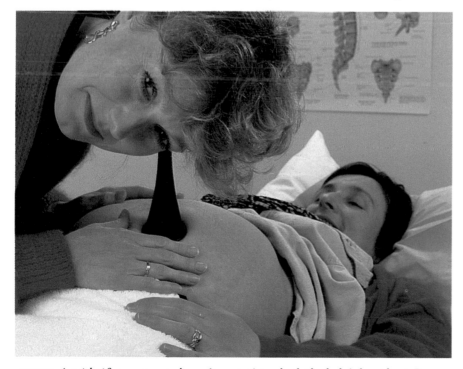

*ABOVE: A midwife uses an ear horn (trumpet) to check the baby's heartbeat. It may seem low-tech, but this piece of equipment is very effective to the trained ear.*

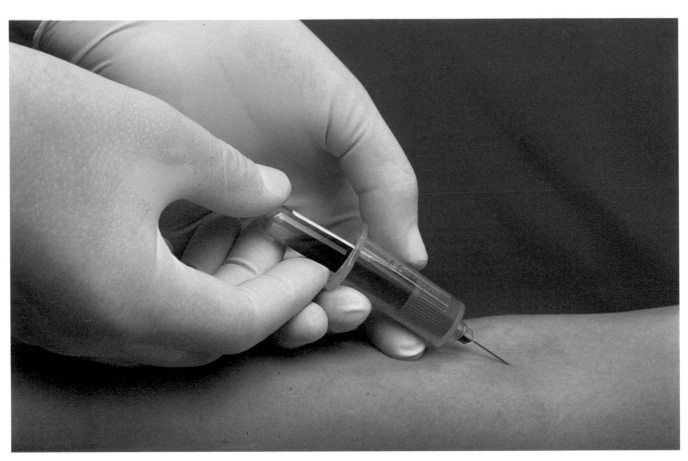

*ABOVE: Taking a blood sample from the mother (the MSAFP screening test).*

### WHAT'S AVAILABLE?

**Maternal Blood Test (MSAFP Test)**

**At**: 16 to 18 weeks.

**Checks**: the Maternal Blood Test, also called the AFP (Alphafoeto-protein) Test or Barts Test, checks AFP levels in the mother's blood. If they are either high or low this can suggest a problem: for example, high levels (a "positive" result) have a number of possible causes, including multiple pregnancy (twins, triplets), a big baby, the baby being older than everyone first thought, bleeding inside the womb and—rarely—structural problems in the foetus, such as kidney or intestinal malformations, chromosomal problems, or some neural tube defects (NTD), such as spina bifida.

**Note**: nine out of every ten women with a raised AFP level do not have a handicapped baby.

**Accuracy**: approximately 90 per cent for spina bifida detection.

**Results**: in about one week.

**Risk**: none.

### Early Ultrasound Screening Scan

**At**: in the UK an early scan may be done at 11 to 13 weeks to scan for size and dates; it also checks the position of the placenta, and the foetus's position and viability.

**Checks**: uses high-frequency sound waves emitted from a hand-held transducer, which is passed over the mother's abdomen, or from a vaginal probe, to build up a black-and-white picture of the baby on a monitor.

This can also be an alternative screening test for Down's syndrome, by checking the size of the space between the back of the foetus's neck and the amniotic sac. If it's 5 mm (¹/4 inch) or more, the risk that the foetus may have a chromosomal abnormality is 25 times greater than usual. If it's less than 3 mm (¹/8 inch) the risk is less than 0.2 times, according to researchers at King's College Hospital, in London. Unless the scan is followed up by a diagnostic amniocentesis test a week or two later, another detailed scan at 20 weeks is still recommended to exclude problems not due to chromosomal abnormalities, such as spinal and/or head problems or limb or major organ malfunctions.

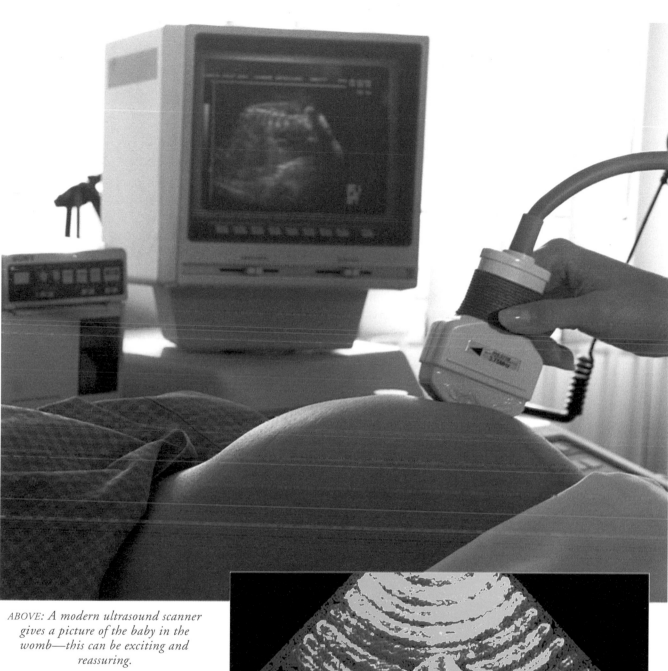

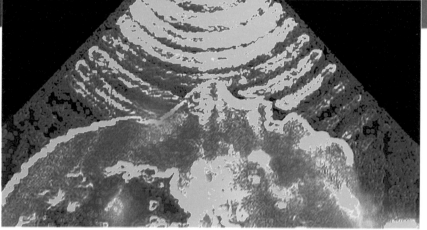

*ABOVE: A modern ultrasound scanner gives a picture of the baby in the womb—this can be exciting and reassuring.*

**Accuracy**: depends on what the radiographer is looking for—with regard to the baby's general development and well-being, accuracy is good. The test will detect between 70 and 80 per cent of major chromosomal abnormalities.

**Results**: immediate.

**Risk**: none.

*ABOVE: Ultrasound is now routinely used to check on the progress of a pregnancy, but some sources suggest that it can give the baby a headache.*

### The Double Test/Triple Test

**At:** 13 to 16 weeks.

**Checks:** this test, also called the Barts Test (see MSAFP Test earlier) or simply "Maternal Serum Screening", is another blood test carried out on you, the mother. It checks either two, or often three, substances. It is an extension of the MSAFP Test (see above), but in addition to checking AFP for neural tube defects, it also checks the level of the hormone human chorionic gonadotrophin (HCG), plus another hormone called unconjugated oestriol. These, together with the mother's age, are used to assess the *likelihood* (only) of Down's syndrome. Results need to be interpreted differently in cases of twin pregnancies, or if the mother has insulin-dependent diabetes.

**Accuracy:** 60 per cent in detecting Down's syndrome.

**Results:** 10 days.

**Risk:** none.

### Amniocentesis

**At:** in some centres of excellence or specialist research units this test is performed early: early amniocentesis may be conducted at 10 to 12 weeks, but 14 to 16 weeks is more common.

**Checks:** a small sample of amniotic fluid, and cultures the stray foetal cells floating in the fluid, to rule out the possibility of Down's syndrome and other major chromosomal abnormalities, or to determine the baby's sex (parents are not always given the last piece of information, however). The fluid, between 7 and 20 ml (1½ and 4 teaspoons), is taken via a fine syringe passed

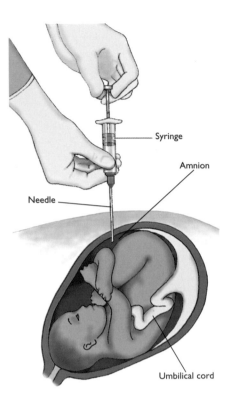

ABOVE: *Amniocentesis is the method used to detect whether a baby is likely to be born with Down's syndrome or other major chromosomal abnormalities.*

through the mother's abdomen and womb wall, guided by ultrasound.

**Note:** after having the test, the mother may need to lie down and rest quietly for a few hours, and some women feel it is best to take it easy for several days. There are not any official guidelines on this.

**Accuracy:** about 99 per cent.

**Results:** 3 to 4 weeks.

**Risk:** there is a small possibility of miscarriage due to the amniocentesis itself (in any case, some confirmed pregnancies miscarry in the first trimester). American sources put it at 0.2 to 0.5 per cent, writes Paul Wexler, Clinical Professor in Obstetrics and Gynecology at the University of Colorado. British figures, from the Harris Birthright

## CORDOCENTESIS

If a detailed ultrasound scan shows up any possible problems, a test called cordocentesis, or umbilical cord sampling, may also be performed. This involves taking a sample of the foetus's own blood with a syringe from the umbilical cord. The cord does not have any nerve endings, so this does not cause the baby discomfort, although there is a 2 per cent risk of miscarriage. The test obtains the same information as amniocentesis, but it also provides important additional data about the baby's state of health in late pregnancy, and can check for foetal infections, metabolic disorders and certain genetic abnormalities, as well as diagnose or treat blood disorders, and assess babies that are "small for their dates". It also checks for Fragile X syndrome, which is sometimes associated with learning disabilities and mental retardation.

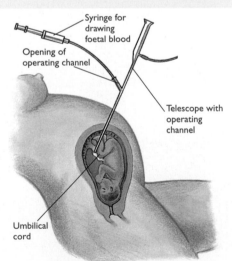

ABOVE: *Foetal blood sampling is sometimes performed to detect certain infections, abnormalities or blood disorders in the unborn baby. The test is called cordocentesis in the United Kingdom.*

Research Centre, in London, are slightly higher: 0.4 to 1 per cent. According to research conducted at the University of Columbia, in Vancouver, Canada, in 1996, early amniocentesis (taken as 11 to 13 weeks) appears no more likely to cause a miscarriage than a later test.

There is also about a 1 per cent risk of severe, unexplained breathing problems for the baby at birth.

**Chorionic Villus Sampling (CVS)**

**At:** CVS can be done as early as 9 weeks, but usually at 11 to 13 weeks. **Checks:** chromosomal abnormalities (as does amniocentesis). Involves removing a small frond of chorion tissue—the fluffy mass of fingerlike projections that surround the fertilized egg, then the early embryo sac, and which later forms the placenta. This grows from the fertilized egg

just as the baby does, so its genetic material is the same. To get the tissue sample, a fine needle is passed through the mother's abdomen and womb, then, guided carefully by ultrasound, it can aspirate off a small section of a villus.

**Note:** there are reports of a small number of limb and/or facial defects through CVS, both in the United Kingdom and the United States.

## POSSIBLE WEIGHT GAIN IN PREGNANCY

Fierce arguments rage among professionals about how much weight women are supposed to put on during pregnancy. Two top London consultant obstetricians, Gordon Bourne and Malcolm Gillard, have drawn up a suggested timetable of what are probably the most precise ideal guidelines available. Don't worry if you put on a bit more than their figures suggest— these estimates are considered to be quite strict. Just eat as sensibly and healthily as you can, as your appetite dictates.

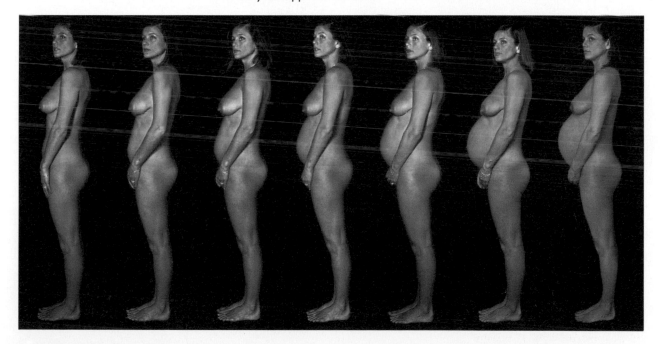

- 0 to 14 weeks: no gain. Some women may even find that they actually lose a bit of weight if morning sickness affects their appetite or they are vomiting.

- 14 to 20 weeks: 3 kg (6.5 pounds).

- 20 to 30 weeks: 5 kg (11 pounds: this is the hardest time to restrict weight gain).

- 30 to 36 weeks: 3 kg (6.5 pounds).

- 36 to 40 weeks: no gain (from week 38 some mothers lose a little weight).

Figures taken from: *Pregnancy* by Gordon Bourne FRCS, FRCOG, revised by Malcolm Gillard FRCS, FROCG (Pan Books, 1995, UK).

According to Professor Wexler, figures vary from 4 in 400 babies to 5 in 10,000. According to Professor Geoffrey Chamberlain, it's less than 1 per cent. The timing of the test, the amount of tissue removed and the tester's skill are all important.

**Accuracy:** 98 to 99 per cent.

**Results:** about 10 days to 4 weeks; sometimes early results in 5 days.

**Risk:** of miscarriage, slight, about 1 to 2 per cent.

### Detailed Ultrasound Scan for Foetal Abnormalities

**At:** performed between 20 and 24 weeks, a detailed ultrasound checks the foetus carefully and assesses the pregnancy in general.

**Checks:** same as for amniocentesis, plus congenital developmental problems with major organ systems, such as the kidneys.

**Accuracy:** good, but the accuracy varies depending on what's being investigated: for example, congenital malformations of the heart or kidneys. You can obtain specific details from your consultant ultrasonologist.

**Results:** some immediate, while some require specialist consultation and analysis.

**Risk:** none.

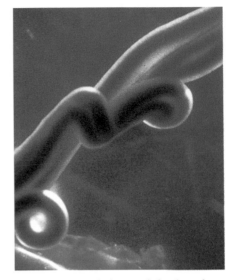

*ABOVE: Your baby's umbilical cord is vital to its well-being.*

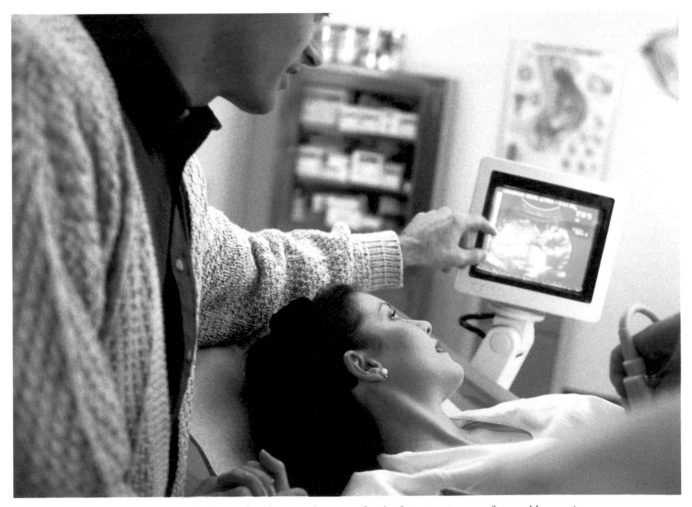

*ABOVE: Seeing your baby on the ultrasound scanner for the first time is an unforgettable experience.*

## WHAT YOUR BABY MAY NOTICE DURING ANTENATAL TESTS

Expectant parents have always been told that their unborn babies would be unaware of the foetal tests being carried out on them. There are now a small number of studies and many anecdotal reports, however, which suggest that ultrasound might cause babies some discomfort (this is especially relevant if you are being offered several scans) and that amniocentesis may, in fact, alarm them.

### AMNIOCENTESIS

Scattered reports and studies suggest that in some cases unborn babies notice the needle, whether their eyelids are still fused (as they are between weeks 10 and 26) or not. Foetuses have reacted with both alarm and aggression to this unknown invader in their territory. Studies published in the *British Journal of Obstetrics and Gynaecology* in 1976 and in the *British Medical Journal (BMJ)* in 1977 (see p. 152) reported varying reactions suggesting alarm, including an accelerated heart rate, slower breathing movements for up to two days afterwards, and remaining motionless for two minutes after the needle had been inserted.

Here are some other examples: one 24-week-old foetus viewed on ultrasound during late amniocentesis was accidentally hit by the needle, and was filmed twisting away and then repeatedly striking out at the needle barrel (*American Journal of Roentology*, 1978); a specialist performing foetal surgery reported he was just about to put a needle into the relevant foetal vein when a tiny hand came up and knocked it away (*British Journal of Obstetrics & Gynaecology*, 1987, UK); Italian researchers Ianniruberto and Tajani described in 1981 a foetus retracting a limb or turning from head to foot when accidentally hit in the arm or in the trunk by a needle. Dr. David B. Chamberlain tells of friends who watched in disbelief as their 16-week-old foetus attacked the needle barrel as it

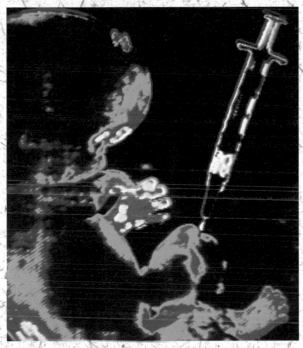

*ABOVE: There is much debate over how much the foetus can feel during antenatal tests, such as the foetal blood test pictured above.*

entered the womb during amniocentesis. On a second try, it again batted the needle away, leaving both the husband and the obstetrician in a cold sweat. The mother said afterwards she had no idea a foetus could do such a thing. Finally, at Queen Charlotte's Hospital, in London, in 1996, foetal medicine expert Professor Nicholas Fisk found an unborn baby's catecholamine (chemicals produced as a response to stress) levels rose after an amniocentesis test.

### ULTRASOUND

In 1975, a study of scanning unborn babies using Doppler ultrasound was published (by H. David et al.) in the *BMJ*.

The researchers didn't tell the mothers whether the scan machine was switched on, but when it was, the foetuses were found to move about much more. In the United Kingdom, in 1993, the Association for Improvement in Midwifery Services' journal, the *AIMS Quarterly*, published a selection of comments from mothers about their babies' responses to being scanned. They included:

"The baby was moving around so much the technician could not take any measurements..."

"It had both hands up to its ears, fist fashion."

"The gynaecologist got very frustrated because he could not get a clear picture because she (the baby) would not sit still. At first she would move to a totally different part of my womb, then when she was bigger, turn around and around."

"She (the baby) was extremely active when we wanted a picture of her. Then she put her head as low as possible in my pelvis where the ultrasound seemed to have difficulty getting a clear picture."

The National Childbirth Trust, in the United Kingdom, received similar information from its members in 1985. Here's one example:

"The scan seemed to upset the baby... it moved and thrashed violently the whole time..."

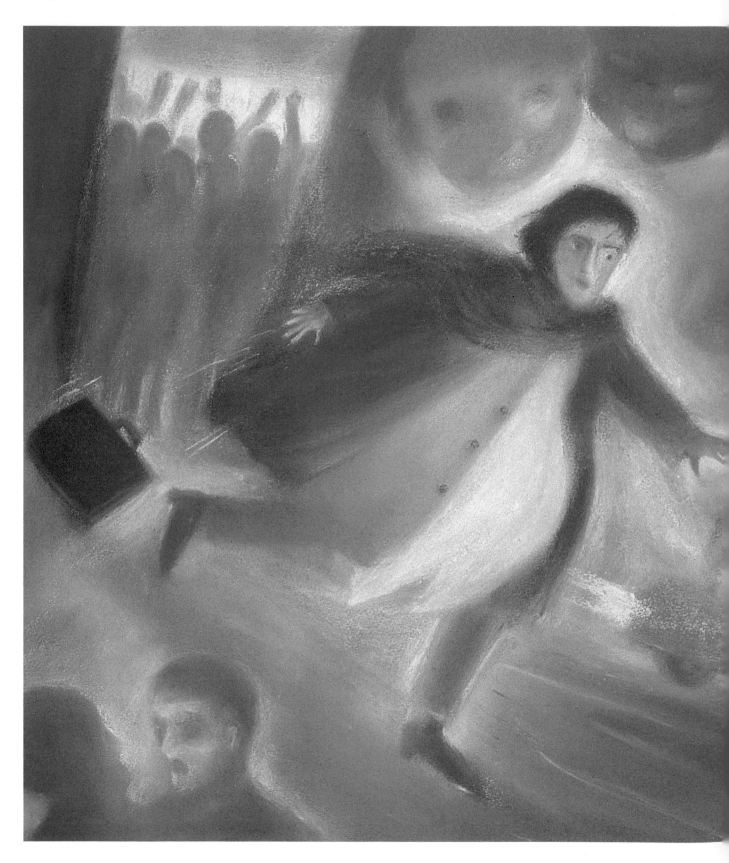

# Does Your Unborn Baby Feel Your Emotions?

## Pregnant women and their unborn babies are arguably in very close emotional and spiritual communication.

Research conducted in 1992 by Dr. David Cheek, an obstetrician in San Francisco, observing 1,000 subjects under hypnosis, strongly suggests mothers and their unborn babies communicate without words, noting "foetal channels for information are psychic (telepathic and/or clairvoyant) and possibly hormonal". According to another American study, in 1995, by a researcher called Dobrovolsky, under hypnosis a group of 25 out of 26 mothers could tell whether their early foetus was a girl or boy. In addition, a report published in *The Pre- and Perinatal Psychology Journal* says that "Unborn babies themselves are quick to pick up on their mothers' thoughts: just one example of many is that babies are more active when their mothers are awaiting ultrasound for an amniocentesis test than when waiting for ordinary ultrasound." So the short answer to the question of whether or not your unborn baby feels your emotions is "yes", because you are both physically inhabiting the same body.

### MOTHER'S INTUITION

This may not be surprising news to many pregnant women. Most mothers have tried talking to their unborn babies either out loud or in their heads, feeling they are often heard and understood when they do so. Most also feel intuitively that being calm is best for the baby that is developing inside them. The ancient Chinese and Japanese believed this, too. They used to conduct prenatal programmes for mothers-to-be—especially those mothers of noble birth—and tried to make sure that the pregnant women only looked at lovely things, heard only beautiful, gentle sounds, and spoke no abusive words. Even today, posters in modern Chinese villages remind pregnant women of this.

### SHARED EXPERIENCE

While your baby develops inside you, he or she is a part of you, feeling most of what you feel and experiencing what you experience. These events may leave a permanent imprint, both psychologically and physically. If you feel relaxed, calm, and happy, so does your unborn baby. For example, in experiments which asked pregnant women to listen to their favourite relaxing piece of music, researchers found the foetuses' breathing movements slowed. In 1990, Dr. Van den Bergh, a Belgian clinical psychologist at the University of Leuven, carried out a study of 70 women pregnant for the first time. By tracking the foetuses' movements and heartbeats to see how they responded when their mothers were under stress, she came to the conclusion that: "Maternal state anxiety... was significantly correlated with foetal behaviour." This was also well illustrated by an experiment at the University of New South Wales, in Sydney, Australia, in 1994, in which pregnant women watched some particularly unpleasant scenes from a Hollywood film. After 20 minutes' viewing time, the foetuses began kicking and their heart rates went up. Violent films and videos drive pregnant mothers from cinemas; and deafening rock music has produced such violent infant kicking that the mothers' abdomens have actually been bruised and their lower ribs broken.

## CHANGING ATTITUDES

"Time in the womb is not a free period for which there are no consequences for anything. The child is already forming its attitudes and its understanding of life from the stimulation that it receives in there"—that's according to Dr. David B. Chamberlain, who is the President of the Association for Pre- and Perinatal Psychology and Health (APPPAH).

We've come a long way from regarding a foetus as what the French philosopher Jean-Jacques Rousseau once brutally described as a witless tadpole. Within the developing field of research into foetal awareness, what has been studied most, apart from the foetus's ability to react to sound, is how a pregnant woman's stress levels affect her unborn baby. There is a large amount of published clinical

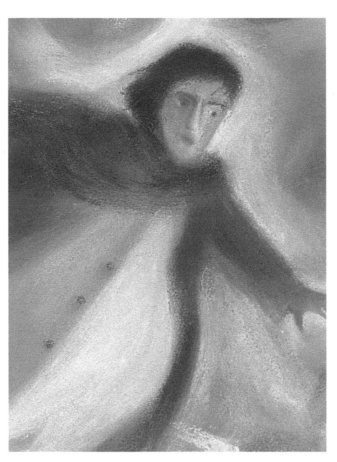

research about this (see p. 152), but it is diverse and fragmented—ranging from studies suggesting that highly stressed pregnant mothers have a greater chance of having a "difficult", irritable baby, who sleeps poorly and regurgitates milk more than most, as well as a greater likelihood of having the baby prematurely. Other studies link stress with smaller head size and poorer brain development, a higher likelihood of congenital birth defects, and a greater possibility of developing psychological problems, such as schizophrenia, later in life. No one knows why this is, although it is thought stress hormones can act as vasoconstrictors, reducing the mother's blood flow, and thereby affecting the vital oxygen and nutri-

ent supplies to the baby across the placenta. It is also possible that maternal stress hormones could have a detrimental effect directly on the foetus's developing neurological system.

## WHAT YOU CAN DO

Some of this information may sound alarming, especially if life during your own current or previous pregnancies has been tough or tiring. So it is not surprising that the immediate reaction of most mothers to the news of foetal sensitivity is worry and guilt: "What have I done? Those arguments we had... the major upheaval of moving... working hard up to the last minute of pregnancy to safeguard my job... getting so tired and cross... have I harmed the baby?" Stop! You did the best you could at the time—remember?—and you could hardly have acted on information you did not even have then. The major up-side to all this is that although this sort of information cannot help you change the past, it empowers you to deal differently with the future—a bright future which includes both enhancing your baby's years of infancy and childhood and a new approach to any future pregnancies.

If your baby has already been born following a stressed pregnancy, you can help now by providing all the love, happy stimulation and care he or she needs. And, while your baby may not show signs of any problems related to life in the womb, keep half an eye open for anything that could be included in what Professor Hans Lou, of Denmark's John F. Kennedy Institute, calls "foetal stress syndrome". This can include a variety of difficulties, some minor and some major, ranging from a barely noticeable mild attention-deficit disorder and left-handedness (see p. 62), to problems such as chronic insecurity or learning difficulties. This way, if there is anything requiring help, the quicker you spot it, the more successfully you can support and encourage your child in dealing with it.

### THE SECRETS OF A POSITIVE PREGNANCY

Unless circumstances are very difficult, there is nothing complicated about this advice and anyone can enjoy—or at least experience uninterrupted stretches of—a happy and positive pregnancy. You do not have to be calm from week 1 to 40. Problems do occur and there are

stressful events which may be impossible to avoid in any woman's life, whether she is pregnant or not, but the trick is not to let stress become constant or chronic.

Knowing that your baby feels what you feel does not mean that you need to talk to him or her inside the womb all day, avoid all differences of opinion with other people at any cost, have long, in-depth relaxation and bonding sessions each morning while listening to special (and often expensive) foetal stimulation tapes, swim with dolphins, meditate upon or pray for your child for several hours every day or, indeed, do anything at all that is special or out of the ordinary.

### BE GLAD ABOUT IT

According to Dr. Thomas Verny, a Toronto-based prenatal psychology expert (Founding President of the APPPAH), one of the best things a mother can do—apart from trying

to remain calm, which is often easier said than done—is to want her baby, and to be looking forward to the birth, as the unborn child will be powerfully aware of the way she feels towards him or her. Unborn babies seem to know when they are wanted, and this forms the foundations they need to feel happy and secure in their life ahead. Sadly, the opposite is also true. According to Czechoslovakian research in 1988, children born to those mothers who tried unsuccessfully to abort their unborn babies have a higher level of psychological problems later. An American study of 8,000 middle-class new mothers, in 1994, also found that unwanted babies were nearly $2^{1}/_{2}$ times more likely to die within their first month of life than those who were wanted.

### RELAX REGULARLY

Whether you choose to put your feet up and listen to gentle music for even 15 minutes a day or go swimming three times a week, you have double the excuse now that you know it really does benefit your baby as well as you. If you have a stressful job, you are fully justified in asking for some of the pressure to be taken off you, to have more temporary help, or to be moved to less-demanding tasks for a while. If you'd like to move to have more space for your baby (and the second half of pregnancy is a very popular time to move), consider, if at all possible, doing it a year or so after the birth rather than in the last few months before, because moving scores high on stress tables. You also have a cast-iron excuse to ask people not to upset you, and for avoiding major arguments.

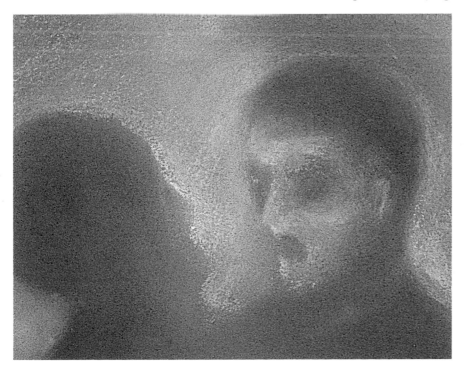

## DEAL WITH ANY GUILT

Try not to nurse guilt about any past pregnancy stress you may have had. "Feeling guilty is a natural reaction to understanding the reality of foetal awareness for the first time," says Dr. Chamberlain. "Yet, it's not a question of how ignorant someone has been, but how enlightened they can be, and how they try to do things differently when they know the facts. There is no escaping the reality of foetal sentience. But guilt is something you can escape from because you do it to yourself.

"It is true that our society has created a lot of expensive problems stemming from prenatal trauma. Such problems demand expensive repair in the form of years of psychotherapy, which because of its cost is not readily available to everyone. We need to change the way we handle pregnancy and birth because foetuses are very sensitive and are learning from experience in the womb. They are not passive bystanders, nor are they just growing organs. They are also growing and developing responses. If they receive a lot of stress stimuli their neurological and endocrine systems will be set at a certain level (i.e., to expect stress, and therefore be modified to survive in a scary environment), and it is very hard to reset these later in life—so these children will grow up to overreact to situations.

"But the opposite can also happen. To feel calm in the womb and sense their mother's relaxation and balance steadily builds up trust and security, just as it should be between mothers and their children."

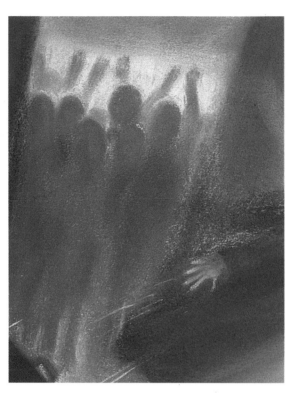

## CRUCIAL TIMES FOR CALM

There are certain times when it is especially beneficial for the mother to remain calm. The first ten weeks are when the baby's major organs and body systems are forming. In the second trimester, the parts of the brain related to memory and adjustment are developing. And towards the end of pregnancy, the baby's awareness is approaching newborn levels.

## HOW DOES MY STRESS AFFECT MY BABY?

There are some experts in prenatal development, such as the paediatrician Dr. Vivette Glover, at London's Queen Charlotte's Hospital, who maintain that when a mother is upset, her blood pressure changes, so that pressure of the blood flowing through the placenta to her baby drops, thereby reducing the vital food and oxygen supply, and that

this causes the foetus long-term problems. Most prenatal psychologists would disagree, however, believing the true cause of such problems to be the hormones the mother naturally produces under stress.

Stress is still seen by many as an overused term, although it describes a clear set of chemical consequences of stimuli, and its effects have been well documented in many areas of medicine from immunology to labour pain. Its effects on unborn human babies are traditionally difficult to prove: the type of clinical experiments required could be cruel to conduct, so much of the work relies on animal studies using rats and mice. Yet, in 1997, according to Peter Hepper, Professor of Foetal Medicine at Queen's University in Belfast, Northern Ireland, there was a huge body of research into all the short- and long-term effects of maternal stress on babies, and the children and adults they grow up to be. Basically, the mother/foetal stress transmissions system works, according to Dr. Lee Ellis, of Minot State University, in the United States, because maternal stress hormones such as cortisol, adrenaline and corticosterone, cross the placenta. Once they get there, these chemical messengers stimulate the foetuses' own fight/flight responses, and also interfere with their production of sex hormones, especially testosterone (hence the connection between a stressed pregnancy and a left-handed baby—handedness is influenced by testosterone levels).

As to whether foetuses are sufficiently well developed to experience

## STRESS—THERE'S MORE OF IT ABOUT

Towards the end of the 20th century people are having to cope with greater levels of stress—at home and, increasingly, at work.

"Stress is a growing issue in pregnancy, because levels have doubled since 1985," says Dr. Nicholas Hall, Director of the University of South Florida Psychiatry Center in Tampa, Florida, "especially in Britain, where one in 59 workers puts in a 70-hour week—that's even more than Japan."

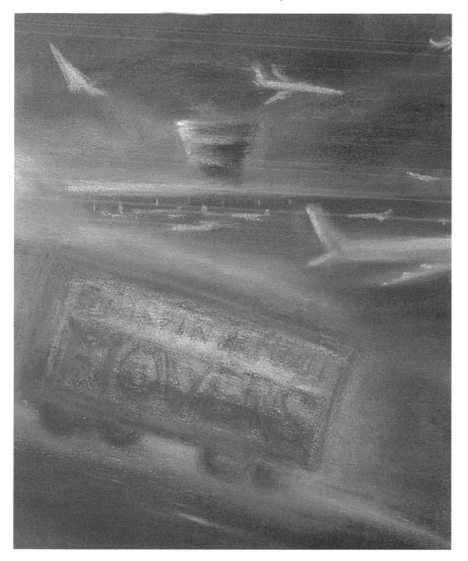

what we understand as "stress", British expert Dr. Alan Watkins says: "Stress exists independently of the cortex, the thinking part of the brain." If thinking's not involved, this also suggests a foetus can suffer from stress transmitted from the mother at a very early stage of development in the womb, while the brain is still at a comparatively rudimentary stage.

Prenatal psychologists and progressive obstetricians think that it is the possible flooding of an immature foetus's system with "alarm/alert" hormones that may produce a consistent state of over-alertness and reactivity similar to an adult in a stressful situation, but with no outlets for it, like a taxi driver permanently stuck in inner-city traffic jams. "The foetus's developing system organizes itself around the environment it finds itself in. If it attunes itself to a repeatedly stressful uterine environment, it will be physically and neurologically primed to be this way outside the womb as well," explains Dr. Chamberlain. This gives "an edge to the selection of stress-related circuits," as Christopher Vaughan, a biochemical sciences editor of Cambridge University Press, in the United Kingdom, puts it.

### LONG-TERM EFFECTS

Being constantly awash with these chemical alarm signals seems to have two possible consequences for a foetus. According to studies of stressed female rats, they produce babies whose "responses were more slow and... who showed more 'emotionality' all through their adult life". This is backed up by several other studies, some of which go back a long time—such as one that was published in the *American Journal of Obstetrics and Gynecology* in 1941 by L. W. Sontag, who found that the whole autonomic nervous systems of babies born to mothers who had been very stressed during their pregnancies were unstable. They showed greater than usual changes in heart rate, their blood vessels were very prone to widening and shrinking and they were also more likely to show rapid changes in their breathing rate—all healthy reactions to sudden stress, but not reactions that should be present all the time.

# The Placenta

The placenta is possibly the most extraordinary
organ produced by the human body, all the more so
because it is temporary.

The placenta was grown, strictly speaking, not by you but by your developing baby to act as a skilled mediator between your two systems. It is arguably the hardest-working organ in your body during this time, and from week 12 it is solely responsible for guaranteeing that your pregnancy remains stable and your baby is not lost in a miscarriage. Perhaps its most impressive achievement, however, is that it manages to remain embedded in your womb wall rather than being rejected by your body, despite the fact that it is technically foreign to your body because it has grown from a fertilized egg containing half your partner's genetic material as well as half your own.

The placenta serves a dual purpose. The tips of the chorionic villi, the frond-like projections on the placenta, dip into lakes of the mother's blood in the wall of the womb lining, passing nutrients, oxygen and often other substances such as hormones into the baby's bloodstream. Conversely, the waste products which the baby needs to get rid of pass back the other way and are eliminated by the mother's system. When the baby is born, the placenta will weigh up to a fifth as much as he or she does.

Some traditional societies call the placenta the tree of life, and many regard it as something supernaturally special. They believe it isn't just vital for the baby's growth and development inside the womb—which, indeed, it is for at least 34 of the 40 weeks—but that it is essential for physical and spiritual growth and development outside the womb, too. Malaysians call the placenta the baby's "little brother". The Minangkabau people believe it should be buried under the front step of the family house, so that however far afield the child travels when grown, he or she will always return home. In the United States, Native Americans have great respect for the placenta, too. A Cherokee father, for example, carries it across two mountain ridges and buries it with special incantations to guarantee a reasonable two years before his wife has another baby. The Thais believe that the placenta should be buried by a

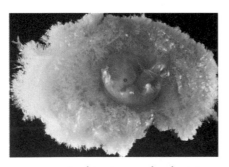

*ABOVE: In this picture, the chorion surrounding a six-week-old embryo has been opened up. The portion at the left will soon give rise to the placenta.*

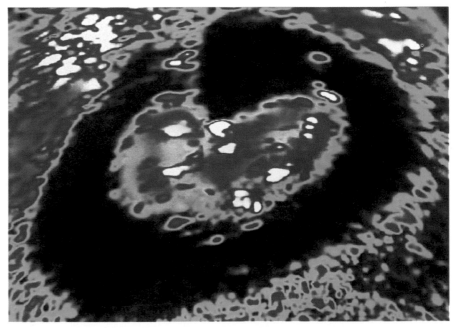

*ABOVE: The placenta (coloured pink) visible in this ultrasound scan of a nine-week-old foetus has formed around part of the amniotic sac. It is a baby's lifeline during the time it spends in the womb.*

water pot so that the baby's heart will remain cool, thus preventing the onset of infant fevers.

Western societies tend to see a placenta more as "the afterbirth"—something rather messy to be disposed of tidily after labour. It is usually either incinerated or sent to drug companies so they can extract and use the rich supply of hormones it contains. Nevertheless, in parts of the United Kingdom and some other European countries, there is a rural tradition that it is beneficial to the health of the new mother to eat the placenta. In anecdotal reports from some women who prefer to give birth at home, and feel that consuming the placenta is a positive and perfectly logical idea, it is recommended that it should be prepared like a piece of liver, fried with garlic and onions. There are other anecdotal reports that to do so can help prevent post-natal depression (PND). However, Professor Channi Kumar, a PND expert at the Institute of Psychiatry, in London, comments: "PND is certainly linked to the massive drop in hormones mothers experience in the first few days after childbirth, but it's unlikely they could absorb the huge amounts in the placenta, which may be denatured by digestive acids and enzymes anyway."

## THE PLACENTA—WHAT DOES IT ACTUALLY DO?

The placenta is the point of contact where your own and your baby's circulatory systems meet but do not mix. In some areas the placenta is only a single cell thick, yet it performs its function as a barrier between the foetal and maternal blood supplies highly efficiently.

Its job involves:
- allowing oxygen, hormones, beneficial antibodies against disease and nutrients to flow through to the developing baby;
- simultaneously screening out most harmful substances;
- channelling your baby's waste products, such as urea and carbon dioxide, which it cannot deal with itself yet, back out again and into your blood supply to be carried off and dealt with by your liver and kidneys.

The placenta certainly works hard. Ten weeks after fertilization, while it still only weighs 50 g (1.8 ounces), it makes about 2 g (0.05 ounce) of protein every day. As if that responsibility and serving as a go-between for your system and your baby's were not enough, it also produces hormones. One of the most important of these is progesterone, the sex steroid which maintains your pregnancy and prevents the foetus from being shed from your womb in the form of a heavy period or, at a later stage, as a miscarriage. Initially, until week 10, the vital progesterone is made by the corpus luteum (the capsule in which your ovary has ejected the ripened egg now developing into your baby). From then on the placenta starts taking over progesterone production, doing so entirely by the 14th week.

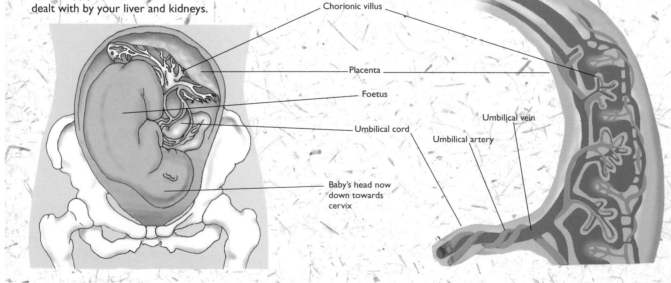

Chorionic villus

Placenta

Foetus

Umbilical cord

Umbilical vein

Umbilical artery

Baby's head now down towards cervix

# You at 16 Weeks

Most women regard the 16-week stage as the beginning of the best part of their pregnancy—the mid-trimester period of months four, five, six and seven. Your morning sickness should have disappeared, your energy will probably have come back (many women report feeling more energetic and creative now than ever before) and two-thirds of women report a major upsurge in sexual desire, too. If you were concerned about miscarriage, the good news is that it is most unusual after the 16-week mark.

Physically your womb has now risen up out of the pelvic cavity. If it was pressing against your bladder before, giving you an urge to urinate frequently, this should not be a problem again until the last two months or so of pregnancy. Because the womb itself has now grown to the size of the average honeydew melon, you will have a small but definite bump, which will reach halfway between your pubic bone and your naval.

Your skin, in general, will be becoming increasingly darkly pigmented, especially if you are a brunette. The linea nigra, the fine dark line which appears down the centre of the abdomen about week 15, will have appeared, and any moles, freckles or birthmarks you have will also darken.

You might also develop "the butterfly mask of pregnancy". This is a darker area of skin colouring spreading over your nose and cheeks and occasionally your forehead like a butterfly's wings. It may be even or blotchy, but usually fades within three or four weeks after having a baby. Cosmetic sunblock can help prevent it developing too markedly if you are in sunshine or strong ultraviolet light.

If you are Caucasian, your facial complexion may be starting to look pinker, partly because of the extra blood volume in your body and partly because all your blood vessels, including those just below the skin, are dilating more easily in response to your rising progesterone levels. This can make a too-pale complexion look prettier and healthier, but is less welcome for someone who has a naturally high colour.

*ABOVE: Sixteen weeks into a pregnancy is often a very reassuring time for women—many say they have more energy than usual.*

The mid-trimester is also the time when you will first feel your baby moving inside you (see Movement— What do Babies do in There?, p. 47). This can be both tremendously exciting and touching, and, along with the return of your energy, the disappearance of nausea, plus a new confidence in the long-term stability of your pregnancy, it all means you will probably be feeling far more positive. Now is the time really to start enjoying your pregnancy and begin looking forward to the birth.

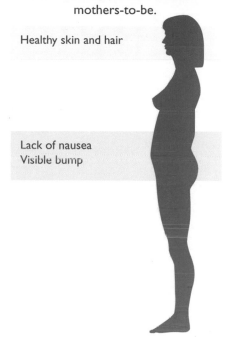

## A TIME TO ENJOY YOUR PREGNANCY

Both physically and mentally, this can be a very positive time for mothers-to-be.

Healthy skin and hair

Lack of nausea
Visible bump

- At 16 weeks you will probably no longer be experiencing the morning sickness of your early pregnancy.

- Your womb, which is the size of a honeydew melon, has risen up out of your pelvic cavity.

Anecdotally, your skin, hair and looks in general are all said to be at their best now (what's known as the traditional "pregnancy bloom"). But don't worry if yours aren't. Blooming isn't nearly as common as everyone thinks it is.

One study published in 1993 in the *British Journal of Obstetrics and Gynaecology* found that out of 375 pregnant women, only a third reported that their hair looked any better than usual.

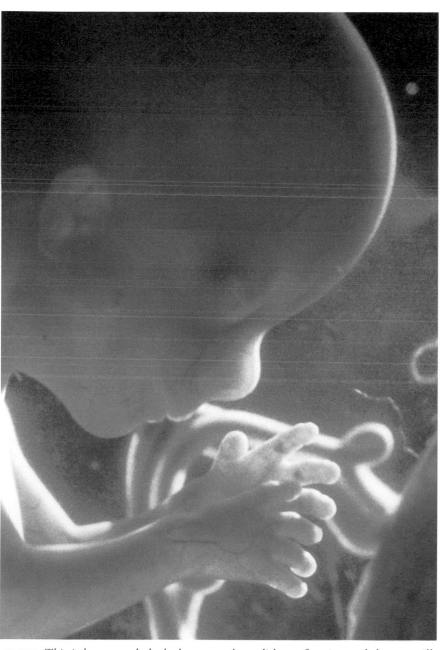

*ABOVE: This is how your baby looks now—the eyelids are forming and the eyes will remain shut for many weeks once complete. The wrists are emerging; the arms, hands and fingers are advancing and developing faster than the legs, feet and toes.*

## GENTLE EARLY STIRRINGS

- At the start of this period unborn babies are 15 cm (6 inches) long and 175 g (6 ounces) in weight.

- By 20 weeks they will have grown to 17.5 cm (7 inches) in length and will have doubled in weight.

Mothers say the first feelings of the baby moving inside them are like butterflies in the tummy, although some, less poetically, just say they thought they were suffering from a case of mild indigestion.

Umbilical cord

Body covered in lanugo

Eyelashes and eyebrows forming

The gentle early movements are most noticeable if you are lying down quietly on your left side, and may be especially so if you have just had some coffee, as the stimulant caffeine crosses the placenta and enters the foetus's own system. Some sugary foods, such as cake, have the same effect because of the glucose they contain.

# The First Movements Mothers Feel

By 17 weeks, your unborn baby is about 15 cm (6 inches) long and weighs 175 g (6 ounces). His or her tiny body is covered in fine, downy hair called lanugo—yet another link with our animal ancestors, but with apes this time, rather than amphibians. This fine hair will usually have disappeared by birth. During the next 3 weeks, your baby will double in weight until an average length of 17.5 cm (7 inches) from crown to rump is

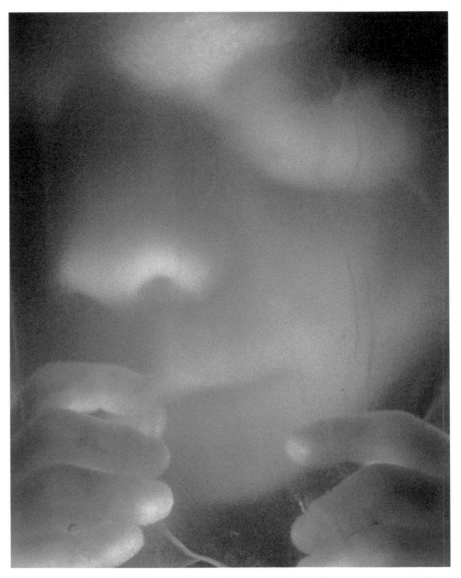

*ABOVE: Babies begin hiccuping at around nine weeks—by the time they reach about seven months, even you can feel it. Bouts can go on for several minutes.*

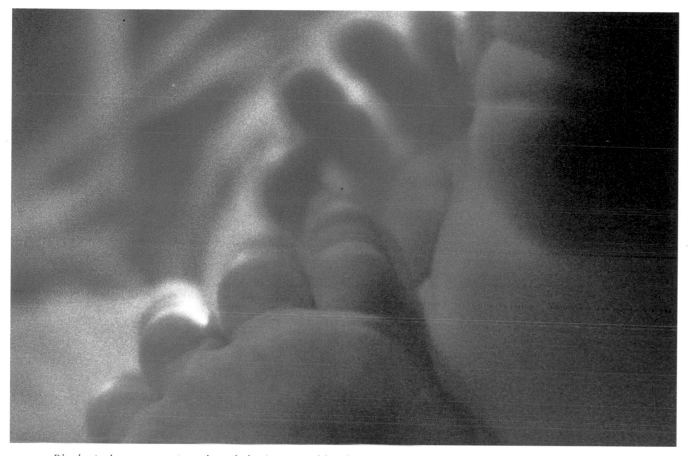

*ABOVE: Rhythmical movements in unborn babies' arms and legs begin at 14 weeks or so. You'll feel them by 16 to 20 weeks, and by the end of the pregnancy the kicks can take your breath away. Partners have even reported being kicked out of bed.*

reached—half the birth length. The head is now one-third of the body size, while the face looks even more human, especially as the eyebrows and eyelashes are beginning to grow.

Foetuses also develop the protective yellow-white waxy and fatty substance called vernix, which covers the skin for most of the rest of their time in the womb. Produced mainly by the sebaceous glands (the manufacturers of the natural oils which keep adult skin supple), vernix sometimes still covers the body at birth, especially if the baby arrives early. Although it may look a bit messy on a newborn baby and it is routinely washed off directly after birth, mothers report that it smells "wonderful".

The spinal cord is gradually covered in a protective sheath of a substance called myelin. If this does not form properly the baby will have neurological difficulties after birth. The links between the muscles and the nerves which activate them are now well established and increasingly used by your unborn baby, so it is not surprising mothers first feel their unborn babies moving inside them during this period. Doctors call this "quickening", and you can now feel your baby kick or roll over because your growing womb has now reached your abdominal wall.

Although the foetus is referred to as such by doctors until birth (and only then does he or she, in clinical

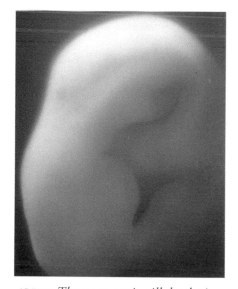

*ABOVE: The outer ear is still developing, but unborn babies begin hearing sounds from outside the womb from just 12 weeks (see p. 97).*

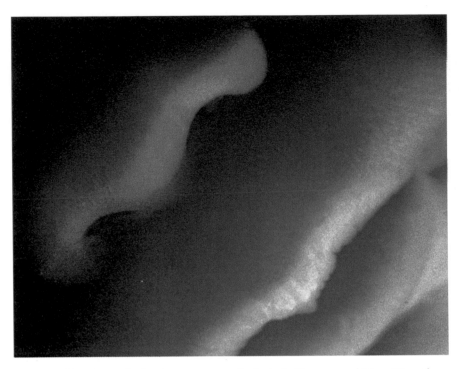

*ABOVE: Yawning and other jaw movements begin in babies at round 11 to 12 weeks.*

terms, become a baby), once a mother has felt her child move it is hard for her to imagine anything inside her other than a baby. Interestingly, Malaysian mothers traditionally believe the 20-week mark is when their unborn babies become fully human—until then they are just said to share their mother's spirit.

Quickening is generally felt between 17 to 20 weeks if the baby is your first, although some mothers say they've detected it earlier, and between 16 and 18 weeks for second and subsequent babies. It may be partly because your womb/abdominal muscles expand faster when they have already been stretched far enough to house a full-term baby before (this is also why first-time mothers' pregnancies tend not to show for longer than those of experienced mothers) and partly because you now recognize the feeling from the last time.

*OPPOSITE: Babies love to play with their umbilical cords—their first toys. The foetus may clutch the cord so firmly that it partly cuts off the oxygen supply coming through it.*

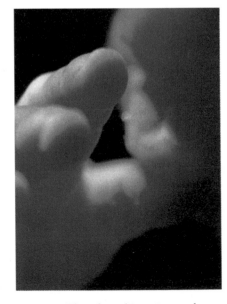

*ABOVE: Thumb-sucking gives unborn babies both soothing reassurance, and, some say, possibly sensual pleasure.*

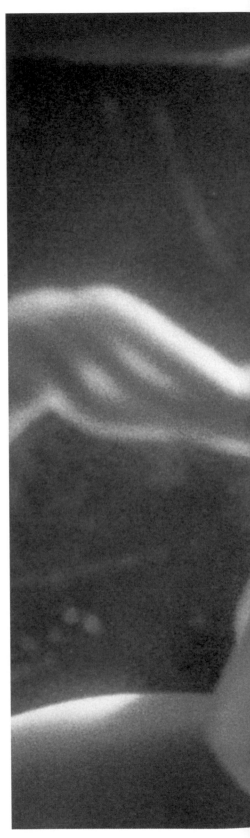

70

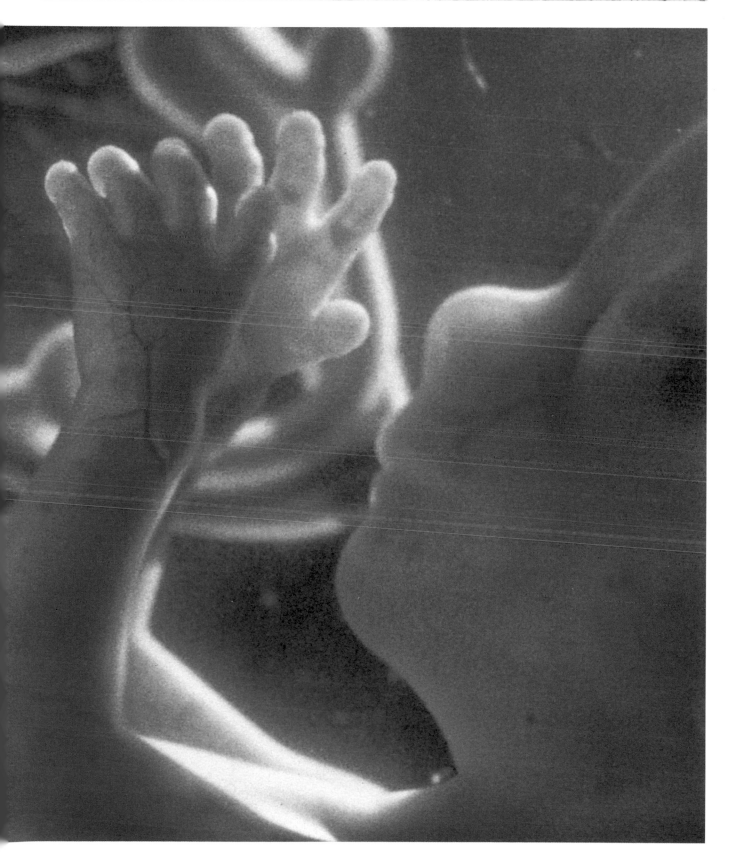

## WEEKS 21–24

### CARING FOR EARLY BABIES

- A foetus born after the 24th week of development stands as much as an 85 per cent chance of survival with the right specialist care.

- The growing foetus is now 20 to 25 cm (8 to 10 inches) in length and about 450 g (1 pound) in weight.

Only a few years ago doctors thought premature babies were not sufficiently neurologically developed to feel pain "as such". Experts now realize that although intensive care for these babies can save their lives, it can also be very uncomfortable.

Hair appearing    Baggy skin

Research has shown high levels of stress hormones such as adrenaline and cortisol in premature babies' bloodstreams. As a result, specialist centres in the United Kingdom and the United States are working to find effective and safe painkillers for premature babies who need specific, often invasive, types of medical care.

# Premature Babies—Tough and Tenacious

At 21 weeks, babies' skin is still thin, with a little fat deposited beneath, so their overall appearance is endearingly baggy, as if they were wearing a diver's wetsuit several sizes too large. Their hearing has now developed enough to recognize the mother's voice—your voice. Teeth buds have formed underneath the gums, and hair is beginning to appear on the head. They can grip with their hands and are often seen on ultrasound holding the umbilical cord.

After 24 weeks, foetuses are sufficiently well developed to have a good chance of survival—up to 85 per cent—if born now, providing they receive expert specialist care,

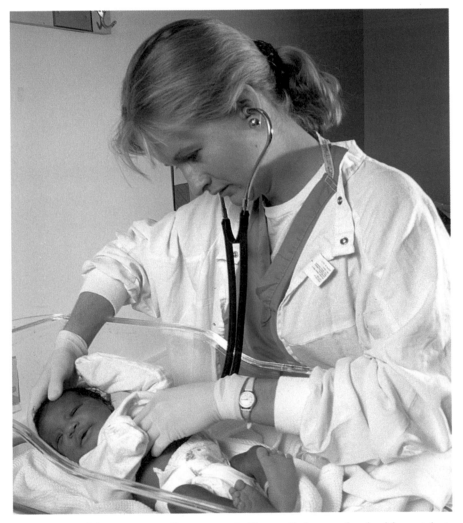

ABOVE: *Careful monitoring of premature babies until they reach a healthy weight is vital in reducing any discomfort or pain they might feel.*

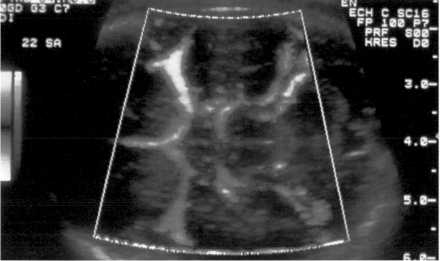

*ABOVE: A scan at 22 weeks can show doctors how well developed a baby is, whether the size is right for the gestational age, or if the baby is "small for dates".*

can-do-it" version of what trained spiritual healers do, and it can work well. Some top British hospitals, such as London's Hammersmith Hospital, employ registered healers in their cancer units; as do some HIV/AIDS centres, such as the Charing Cross Hospital.

Work at the pioneering Queen Charlotte's Hospital, also in London, in 1996, suggests that gently stroking/massaging a premature baby can help lower the level of pain, and carrying a naked baby close to your bare chest—"kangaroo care"—also helps parent and baby, physically and emotionally. Research at the University of Miami Medical School has also shown that when parents stroked their premature babies and moved their limbs gently for only 15 minutes a day, the babies put on 50 per cent more weight and matured faster, plus their hospital stays were, on average, six days shorter.

do not have any major congenital abnormalities and have not suffered any damage to their delicate internal organs during birth. Babies as young as 22 and 23 weeks have also survived and thrived, but this is far less common.

Despite their size—20 to 25 cm (8 to 10 inches) long and 450 g (1 pound) in weight—and apparent fragility, premature babies have repeatedly astonished and delighted their doctors and parents by showing just how tenacious they can be. However, if your baby were to arrive now, he or she would need to be looked after in the special baby-care unit for many weeks. The lungs would not be mature enough to breathe on their own, so the baby would be on a ventilator, and fed through a nasal tube until old enough to take nourishment by mouth.

In the meantime, something vital all parents of premature babies can do to help reduce any discomfort, isolation and distress their babies may feel during special intensive care is to give them very gentle massage and loving

touches. Even holding your hand or hands a little way away from your baby's head, or holding one hand above the baby's forehead and one above the feet, literally "thinking" love and strength into them, can help. It's just a basic "every-parent-

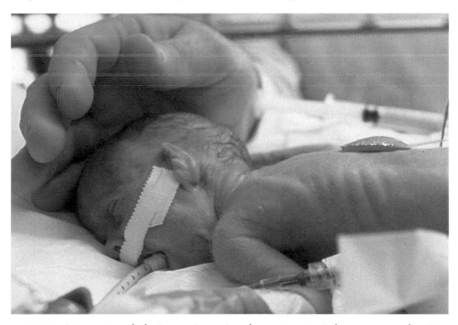

*ABOVE: A premature baby is seen in an incubator at a special care neonatal unit; she is attached to small electrodes that are monitoring her heart rate and breathing, and the incubator itself is keeping her warm. Her father is comforting her with a gentle healing touch—cupping her head without actually touching her.*

## WEEKS 25–28

### CELEBRATING PREGNANCY

- Your unborn baby's taste buds are forming now—he or she will already have developed a sweet tooth.

- Your foetus is now also able to hear music—Mozart and Vivaldi seem to be particular favourites.

Special ceremonies are held around the world to celebrate pregnancy at this time. In Java, for example, the midwife would symbolically break an egg on your sarong to symbolize the opening of your body and to help bring about gentle, easy childbirth.

Taste buds forming

Vernix covering skin

In India, the Pandits have a rite involving "the giving of milk" (in this case yogurt), which is performed by the mother's parents. The ritual is said to guarantee that the mother will be able to breast-feed easily after the birth.

# Why Seven Months is Special

Your baby is now roughly seven months old on the developmental scale, and seven is a number with both magical and spiritual significance for many different cultures around the world, including those in Western Europe and in the United States. In many parts of the world you, the mother-to-be, would now be the focal point of a special ceremony to commemorate and celebrate your seventh month of pregnancy.

The seventh month is also often when parents find they feel secure enough about the stability of the pregnancy to begin gathering baby

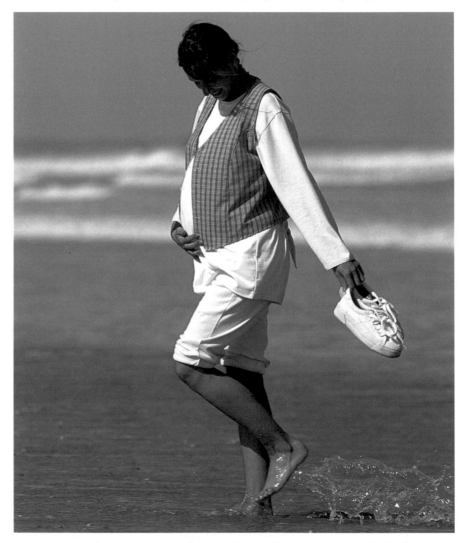

*ABOVE: Try to find time to enjoy this special stage of your pregnancy—do the things you like best. If you can afford the time and money, taking a quiet holiday is a good idea.*

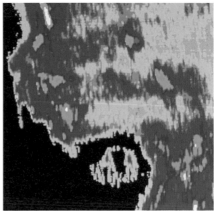

*ABOVE: As shown on this ultrasound scan, at this stage of development, the foetus's profile is clearly visible.*

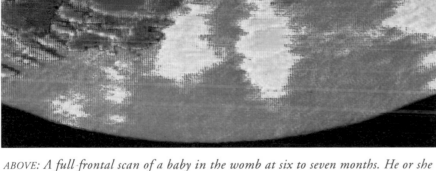

*ABOVE: A full-frontal scan of a baby in the womb at six to seven months. He or she is fully formed and so has a good chance of survival if he or she were to be born toward the end of this period.*

clothes and equipment, as well as decorating the nursery.

At 28 weeks, babies have a very good chance—up to 95 per cent—of survival if born now. However, there is a price tag on premature babies: in countries such as the United States, where the cost is seldom paid by the government (as it is, for example, on the British National Health Service), a stay in a neonatal intensive care unit can cost tens of thousands of dollars, especially if the care lasts a few months.

Your baby will now be up to 30 cm (12 inches) long, and is, because the body has grown more than the head in the past few weeks, almost in proportion; however, he or she still only weighs 1.75 kg (3³/4 pounds). The nostrils have opened as breathing practice is stepped up, with more tiny air sacs called alveoli developing in the lungs. The muscles are becom-

ing well developed, which you will realize only too well as he or she kicks and punches to try them out, sometimes even turning head-over-heels. The skin is now completely covered in vernix to prevent it from becoming waterlogged by its constant immersion in amniotic fluid.

The taste buds are also forming now. Research from as long ago as 1937 showed that if bitter or sweet liquid is introduced into the amniotic fluid, the baby's rate of swallowing decreases—some foetuses have even been seen to be grimacing— or increases, depending on how strongly their "sweet tooth" is developed.

The foetus will also respond to certain stimuli from outside the womb (see What Your Unborn Baby Can Learn, p. 87), for example, remembering and enjoying music. Mozart and Vivaldi appear to be particular favourites (see What Your Baby Can Hear in the Womb, p. 97), according to work by Michelle Clements, a specialist at the International Congress of Psychosomatic Obstetrics and Gynaecology in Rome (1977), and research by Dr. M. Gellrich, published in Hong Kong (1993).

# You at 25 Weeks

Your heart has now enlarged and, to cope with the additional 35 per cent of blood currently flowing in your system, it has to beat an extra 10 times per minute (the usual non-pregnant pulse is roughly 70 beats per minute). That's 14,000 extra beats every day for the rest of your pregnancy. Your womb will be the size of the average pumpkin, having risen three-quarters of the way up your abdominal cavity because your baby is growing rapidly—enough for you to notice you are putting on about 450 g (1 pound) a week, although many mothers-to-be also experience a major growth spurt in the 25- to 29-week period.

As your bump begins to enlarge noticeably, this tends to be the time when you will begin to notice stretch marks appearing on your skin. Estimates vary, suggesting 40 to 80 per cent of pregnant women develop these. They can appear very suddenly, occasionally overnight, as thin bright red lines, and are caused by the elastic fibres below the skin over-stretching and rupturing. Later, scar tissue forms on the site. The red colour fades over the months after delivery, leaving silvery lines instead.

Your breasts might also begin to leak pre-milk (colostrum) now. This is a good sign because it indicates they are getting ready to produce milk so you will be able to breast-feed your baby if you want to. Do not squeeze out any colostrum, however, because this will only stimulate your breasts to make more.

You might also be experiencing some water retention now and notice your ankles and face are a lit-tle puffy. This is quite common. It is partly because the normally high oestrogen levels of pregnancy affect the levels of albumen within the cell tissues, which upsets the cells' salt/potassium balance, causing them to retain more water. It is also partly because of the increased vol-ume of blood and the pressure of your growing baby on certain major blood vessels. To ease puffy feet, legs and ankles, wear Lycra support stockings or tights from the sixth month onward, putting them on before you get out of bed in the mornings, and putting your feet up

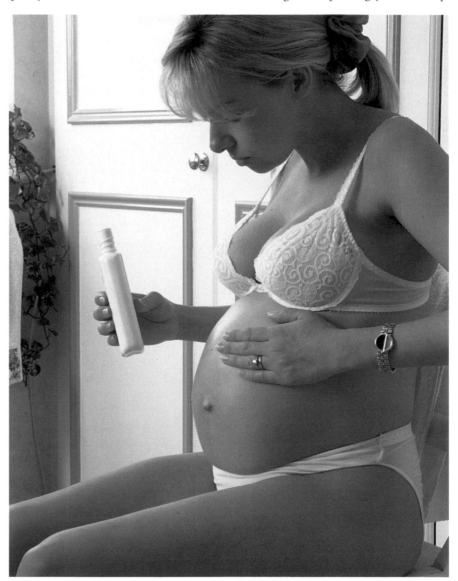

*ABOVE: Stretch marks can appear very suddenly, and there appears to be an inherited link—did your mother or grandmother develop them, for instance? If so, some daily oil-rubbing may help to prevent them.*

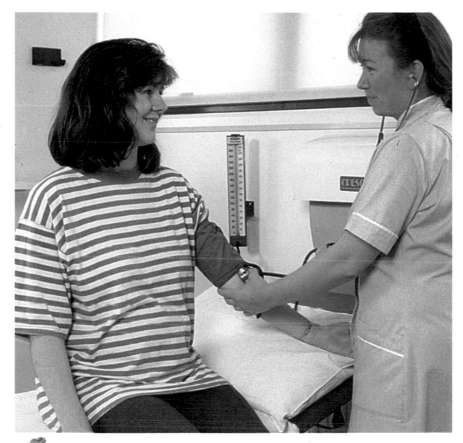

## YOUR PREGNANCY BECOMES MORE VISIBLE

The baby inside you will definitely be apparent to the outside world by now.

Leaking breasts

Stretch marks
Baby's first movements felt ("quickening")

*LEFT: Try to exercise at least three times a week if you possibly can because it really does pay off to be in reasonable physical shape for childbirth.*

*ABOVE: At this stage in your pregnancy, high blood pressure needs to be monitored to rule out pre-eclampsia.*

for a couple of 15-minute periods throughout the day and once or twice in the evening.

If there is a great deal of swelling, your doctor may do a urine test to check for raised levels of protein. These two factors, combined with a sudden rise in blood pressure and headaches, can be a sign of pre-eclampsia, a high blood pressure condition which can occur during pregnancy and requires monitoring, rest and (many experts now suggest) a specific type of diet to help control it. If these measures do not help, you may be admitted to hospital for a while for medical surveillance, complete rest and treatment to lower your blood pressure.

- Your womb is now the size of a pumpkin and your breasts may begin to leak a little pre-milk (colostrum).

- This is the point when, if you are going to develop them at all, you may notice your first stretch marks appearing.

Obstetricians flatly deny anything can be done to help prevent stretch marks. However, Dr. Vivienne Lunny, a former hospital pathologist and now a clinical aromatherapist, as well as a former head of clinical research for the Aromatherapy Organizations Council, in the United Kingdom, suggests a twice-daily massage from the beginning of pregnancy of the abdomen, lower back, thighs and breasts with a mixture of lavender, neroli and mandarin essential oils in a wheat-germ carrier oil can help.

## WEEKS 29–32

### GETTING STRONGER EVERY DAY

- Unborn babies are now starting to develop an immune system.

- They are getting fatter—you can no longer see the network of blood vessels beneath their skin.

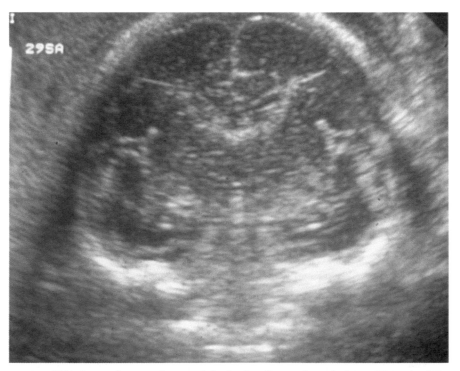

If you are sunbathing with your abdomen uncovered, the light will appear to your baby as a warm orange glow. Babies will even track a light source: if a small torch is moved across your abdomen, your baby will turn to follow the light with his or her eyes and may even try to touch the moving glow.

Eyes open        Increasing fat

Babies in the womb tend to move most often between weeks 30 and 32, because they are now relatively strong and still have plenty of room. At later stages of pregnancy the space they have available is much more restricted and they don't have the same freedom of movement.

# Babies Build up Their Defences

Babies at this stage are perfectly formed, and by week 32 their heads are fully in proportion with their bodies. The eyes, framed by delicately arched eyebrows and a good set of eyelashes, now open once more, so they are able to see the warm red glow of the surroundings and register any strong light.

Unborn babies are now also becoming a little plumper as they are beginning to lay down fat beneath the skin. There are two types of fat in the body: brown fat, which generates heat and which the foetus will need from birth; and white fat, which is an energy source. By week 30, your baby will have produced about 50 g (2 ounces) of fat—3.5 per cent of its total body weight, which will rise to 15 per cent. Although he or she is still thin, you can no longer see the delicate network of blood vessels beneath the skin or the shadowy images of the growing bones.

The building of a defence system against a potentially hostile world is vital to your baby's survival, and he or she is now starting to develop an immune system to fight off germs. For the past few months, the placenta has been taking up some of the antibodies from your bloodstream and releasing them into your baby's

*ABOVE: This is an ultrasound scan of the brain of an unborn baby at 29 weeks. The scan uses high-frequency sound waves to build up an image of soft tissue such as the muscles, organs and brain, and is a good indicator of any problems.*

bloodstream in the last stages of pregnancy. In this way, unborn babies borrow their mothers' immunity to a whole range of diseases until they are able to develop their own. Starting while a baby is still in the womb, this process continues for the first vulnerable weeks and months of life. He or she will receive more of these vital antibodies in the pre-birth milk (colostrum) and breast milk, which will additionally protect against infection during the time it is most vital.

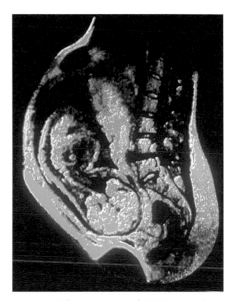

ABOVE: *This is a special NMR (nuclear magnetic resonance) picture of a baby in the womb at eight months of pregnancy. Already he or she has settled into position for birth, with the head touching the mother's cervix at the neck of the womb.*

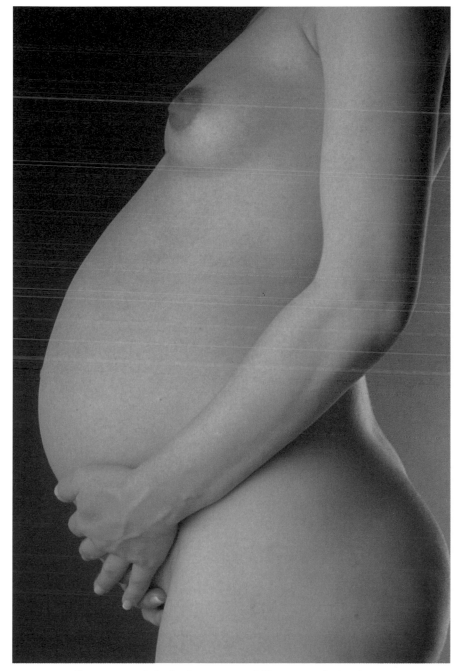

ABOVE: *Every woman's body changes at a different rate during her pregnancy.*

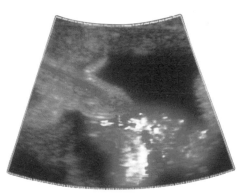

ABOVE: *Babies go through an average 2,400 nappies in the first 2¹/2 years after they are born, and they get plenty of practice passing water in the womb. Here is a scan of a baby boy at 32 weeks, urinating in utero. His body is on the left, his penis at the centre. The small cloud of urine is coloured blueish white.*

## WEEKS 33–36

### GETTING INTO POSITION

• Unborn babies are now about 35 cm (14 inches) in length.

• At this stage they weigh all of 2.5 kg (5¹/2 pounds)— about as much as you might hope to lose on a crash diet in two days.

By now your baby should have turned upside-down with the head pointing downward. For about half of all first-time mothers, this is also when their child's head begins to move down into the pelvis, pressing firmly against the closed cervix (neck of the womb).

Reduced space        Fingernails

When this happens, doctors, nurses and midwives say the baby's head has engaged. Mothers who have had babies before will probably find their baby's head does not engage until the final week of pregnancy, or even as late as the start of labour.

# Preparing for Life Outside the Womb

Your baby has grown so much bigger now—about 35 cm (14 inches) and weighing about 2.5 kg (5¹/2 pounds) at week 33—that he or she is beginning to find it a tight squeeze and will, therefore, probably be moving about less than before. But if he or she stretches or kicks you may see the bump this creates on your abdomen. If a specific bump is the head, foot or hand, you will be able to feel the outline, sometimes quite clearly, with your fingers until the baby shifts position.

Although still relatively thin, your baby is laying down more fat beneath his or her skin and becoming plumper. Tiny fingernails have grown to the end of the fingers, and the toenails will reach the ends of the toes by about week 36 or 37. In boys, the testes should now also be descending from the abdominal cavity down into the scrotum. However, this does not happen in 2 to 3 per cent of cases because of a condition called cryptorchidism (meaning "hidden testes"), which

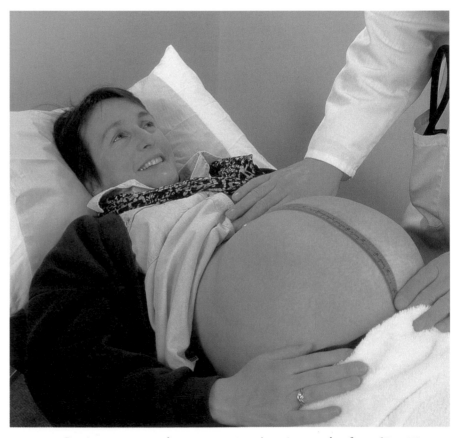

*ABOVE: During pregnancy the average woman's waist stretches from 67 to 70 cm (27 to 28 inches) to 100 to 105 cm (40 to 42 inches).*

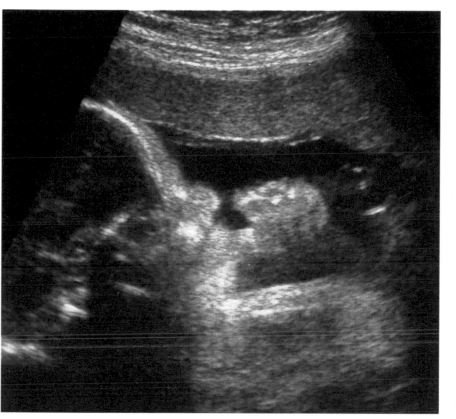

*ABOVE: This picture clearly shows that a baby in the womb at this stage is very well developed—so much so, in fact, that he or she would stand an excellent chance of survival if you gave birth now.*

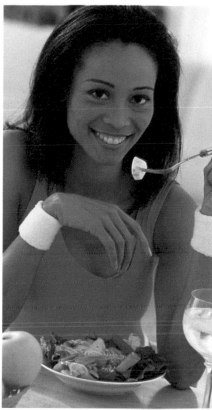

*ABOVE: Eating healthily and feeling good about yourself are essential in adjusting to your ever-increasing size.*

has become three times more common in the West since the 1900s. According to Dr. Richard Sharpe, of the Medical Research Council's Reproductive Biology Unit, in Edinburgh, Scotland, this may be because male babies are exposed to increasing amounts of oestrogen (female sex hormones) in the womb. Scientists at Copenhagen University's Department of Growth and Reproduction also suggest one possible culprit may be the mother's diet, if it has high fat and protein and low fibre contents (the intestine absorbs oestrogen more readily if it only has small amounts of fibre lining it). Another reason could be rising levels of pollution from chemicals,

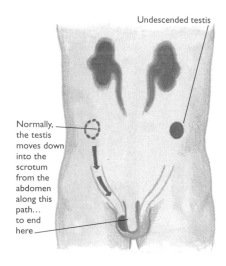

Undescended testis

Normally, the testis moves down into the scrotum from the abdomen along this path... to end here

*Undescended testes (cryptorchidism) is a relatively common condition in which the testes do not descend into the scrotum. Drug or surgical treatment is usually administered.*

such as chlorinated hydrocarbon. Undescended testes need to be corrected with drug treatment or surgery, as they can cause fertility problems later.

For babies born at this stage, the chances of survival are excellent, although they might need help with breathing because their lungs are not yet fully developed. The kidneys are getting plenty of practice for producing lots of wet nappies after birth, because the baby is now releasing about 600 ml (1 pint) of urine daily into the amniotic fluid. The waste products in the urine are filtered through the placenta into your bloodstream and are dealt with by your own kidneys.

# You at 36 Weeks

The movements your baby makes in your womb can now be seen more clearly as rolling undulations and little punching movements pushing out your abdomen. Or you may feel the temporary small, hard protrusions of an elbow or distinct hand or foot shape jammed hard against your womb wall. This is because in months seven to eight the volume of cushioning amniotic fluid has been halved to give your baby more vital growing space.

Your bump will now have reached the base of your rib cage and your navel will have popped outward. Because your lungs have increasingly less room to expand as they are squashed by your growing baby and womb, you may become breathless easily. To relieve this, get down on all fours so your belly hangs away from you, and take a few slow, deep breaths. You may also find you need to urinate more frequently because your bladder will be squashed by your baby's weight and also because of the extra blood flow to your kidneys, which are filtering all the blood in your body thirty times a day. It helps to avoid diuretic drinks, such as tea and coffee, especially at night, but continue drinking other plain fluids (water or milk) to avoid dehydration, and always empty your bladder fully when urinating—lean forward to ensure you pass the last few drops of urine, as any left behind repeatedly can become a breeding ground for infections such as cystitis.

Varicose veins can appear at any point during your pregnancy, but they may be most noticeable in these final weeks. They tend to disappear after delivery, though, because they are caused by the increased progesterone levels of pregnancy relaxing the blood vessels' muscular walls. Because blood is not now being returned to the heart so efficiently it

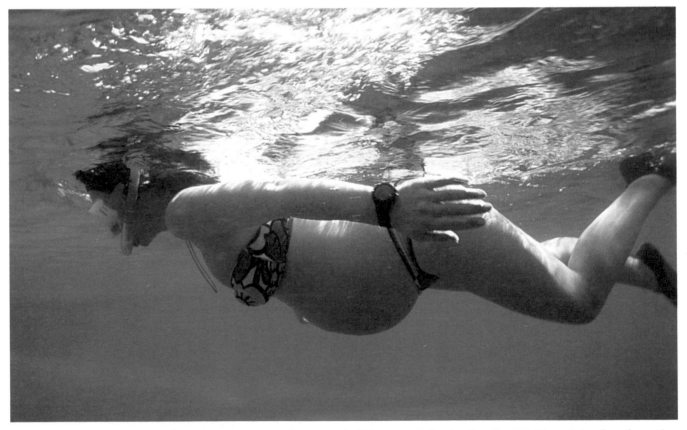

*ABOVE: Exercise is important during pregnancy. According to top British osteopath Stephen Sandler: "It's like training for a five-mile race. If you are reasonably fit you'll sail through it. If you're not, you'll be lucky to get halfway round the course without collapsing."*

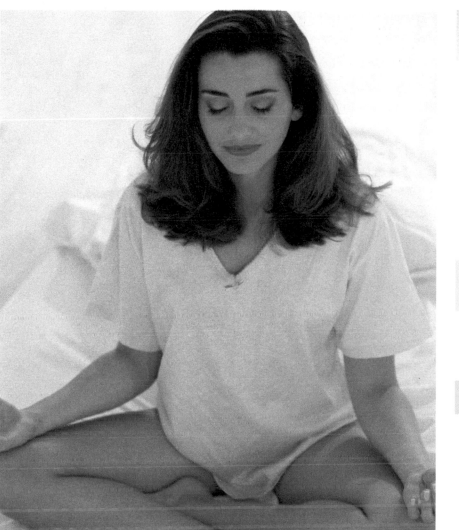

*ABOVE: Practising breathing techniques before birth is a good idea because the more often you do them, the more easily, quickly and effectively they will work for you when it comes to the point that you need them most.*

## A TIME TO SLOW DOWN

At this time mothers-to-be may be starting to feel nervous—and understandably so. But staying patient and calm is important.

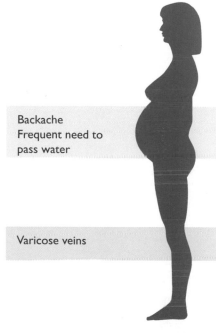

Backache
Frequent need to pass water

Varicose veins

- You may suffer from backache now, even if you did not earlier in your pregnancy.

- Don't worry too much if you develop varicose veins towards the end of your pregnancy—they usually disappear after the birth.

tends to pool in certain areas, distending the blood vessels. The extra 50 per cent volume of blood in your body does not help either, and your baby's head may also be pressing against certain major vessels. Useful measures to help reduce varicose veins include wearing support tights, putting your feet up for 15 minutes every hour, especially in the evening, and regular swimming.

As your pregnancy reaches its heaviest time, you may find you now experience backache if you haven't already. It helps to have some low back massage, to support your belly and back with pillows when lying in bed, and to support your back with a small pillow while you place a pile of books about 12.5 cm (5 inches) high under your feet when you are sitting down. To relieve aching, lie down on the floor, your head supported by a pillow and your legs at right angles to your body lying up and over a chair.

If you are having your first baby, you may now notice a phenomenon known as "lightening". This is when your baby's head engages—moves down deep into your pelvic cavity, thus lowering the level of the top (fundus) of your womb—leaving you temporarily more comfortable breathing-wise. In women who have had a baby before, this does not occur until the 40th week, or sometimes not until the start of labour itself.

## WEEKS 37–40

### YOUR "BABY DUE" DATE

• If you have a delivery date it's probably wrong—you should allow for two weeks' leeway on either side.

• Your unborn baby will no longer kick much, as there is not much room, but will make squirming movements as he or she tries to stretch in the confined space that's left.

The ideal, textboook pregnancy is meant to last for 280 days—40 weeks—measured from the first day of your last normal menstrual period. Another way doctors calculate the date of birth is by setting it 266 days from the date of conception.

Fully formed foetus

While some mothers have no idea of when conception might have been, others say they can pinpoint it exactly and intuitively because they had clearly identified the point at which they ovulated during that cycle.

# Birth Approaches and the Countdown Begins

**B**abies usually arrive any time from now onward. At 37 weeks, they will be about 40 cm (16 inches) long and weigh more than 2.7 kg (6 pounds); by 40 weeks, they are about 50 cm (20 inches) long crown to heel and weigh 3.15 to 4 kg (7 to 9 pounds), sometimes more. This is quite an achievement: your child is 7 times taller than at 12 weeks, and nearly 200 times heavier. There is now very little room for manoeuvre

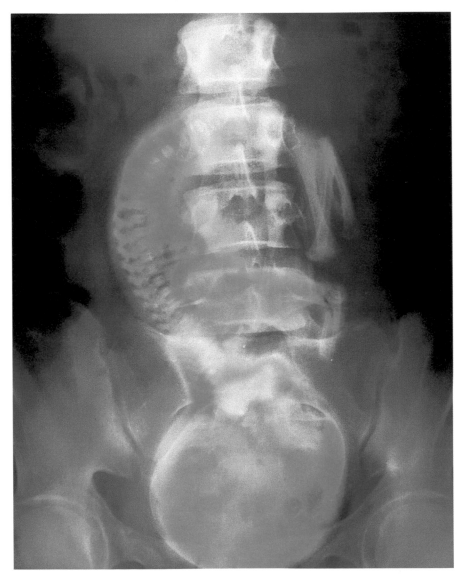

*ABOVE: This coloured X-ray picture shows a full-term foetus positioned ready for birth, facing downward with the head engaged in the mother's pelvic cavity.*

in the womb, so you may feel a pair of small feet pressed hard up against your diaphragm under your ribs, and the occasional energetic kick can take your breath away. Close-to-term babies tend to make vigorous squirming movements as they try to stretch not only their arms and legs but the spine, too, in the confined space. In this last four-week period they put on about 1 per cent of their weight (about 28 g [1 ounce]) daily.

At this point you will probably be wondering when your baby is going to arrive. Delivery dates are based on the average length of women's menstrual cycles, generally supposed to last for 28 days. According to Professor Geoffrey Chamberlain, former President of the Royal College of Obstetrics and Gynaecology, in Britain, however, only 8 per cent of women actually have that typical, clockwork cycle. Firm "baby due" dates also assume babies themselves are ready on time, like preset alarm clocks. They're not. According to Professor Chamberlain. "Only about 5 per cent of babies actually arrive on the day they were expected to, and anything between 38 and 42 weeks' stay in the womb is regarded as normal. Think of your due date as a guideline only and have a due week or even a due couple of weeks in mind instead."

By now your baby looks well-rounded, the skin tone is good and healthy, and most of the fine downy lanugo hair has disappeared from the body. If any remains it is usually around the shoulders, arms, or legs, and sometimes the forehead, but that vanishes completely within a few days of birth. The hair on his or her head is from 1 to 3.5 cm ($1/2$ to $1^1/2$ inches) long. There will proba-

bly still be some vernix in the creases of the body, such as the groin, elbow, neck, and armpits. At this stage, all Caucasian babies' eyes are blue. If your baby is to have eyes that are not blue, the colour may change within a few minutes after birth from blue to the colour—green, brown, grey, hazel—he or she will keep forever.

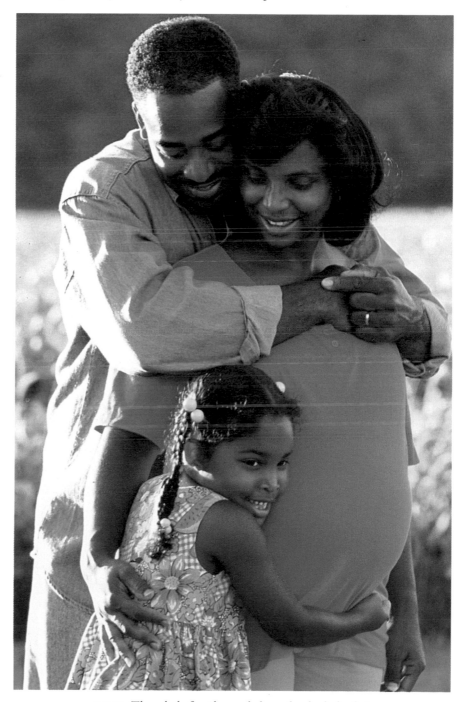

*ABOVE: The whole family can help make the baby feel welcome before he or she is born.*

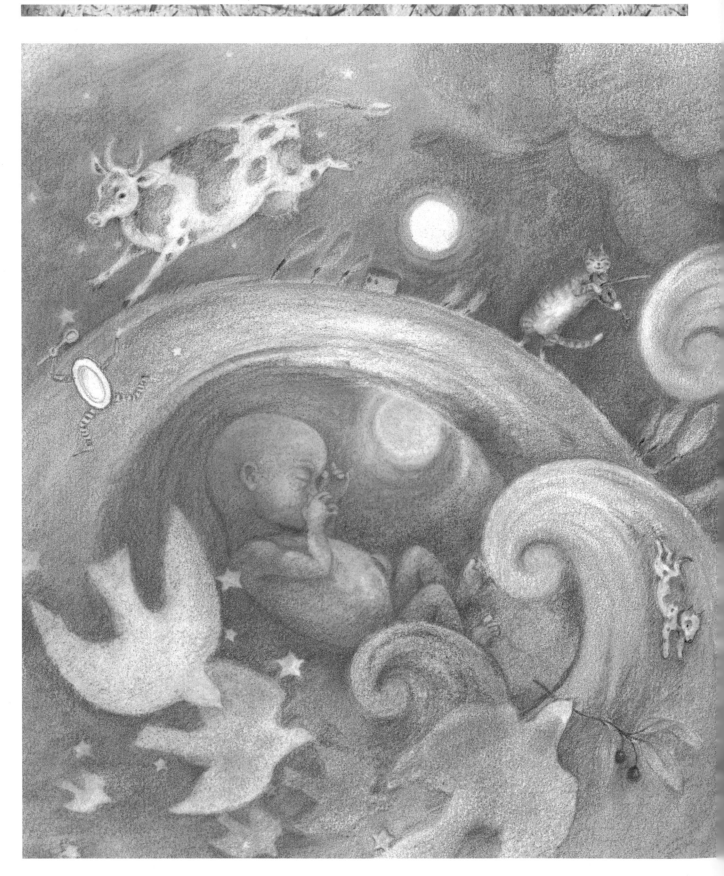

# What Your Unborn Baby Can Learn

Life inside the mother is highly stimulating for babies, who are anything but "asleep" for their nine months' gestation.

Babies up to one year old have been hailed as the most powerful learning machines in nature, because of the rate at which they absorb and assimilate information. Research-based evidence which has emerged over the past 15 to 20 years suggests the womb is a place of intense activity and learning, as well as the place where the baby's physical body, its complex systems and organs, sensory perception and intelligence are being continually formed and refined.

### THE LIMITS OF LEARNING

*In utero*, foetuses learn the early principles of language from hearing their mothers' voices (see What Your Unborn Baby Can Hear, p. 97, and reference, p. 75). Research under hypnosis into prebirth memories suggests they develop memory as well, because so many children and adults have surprisingly accurate spatial and emotional recall of their time in the womb and their own birth (see Memories of Being in the Womb—and Being Born, p. 121, and references, p. 136). Other major studies illustrate effective telepathic communication between mothers and their unborn babies (see Does Your Unborn Baby Feel Your Emotions?, p. 59). Unborn babies can be taught to recognize specific songs and stories, too. In 1994, a team of French and American researchers asked mothers to recite a

nursery rhyme aloud three times a day for a month, between their 33rd and 37th weeks of pregnancy. When researchers monitored the babies' heart rates in the 37th week—three weeks before birth—they responded differently to rhymes they had heard before and rhymes they had not.

During the past 25 years, there has been a number of prenatal development-enhancement programmes demonstrating that it is possible to teach, stimulate and communicate with foetuses *in utero*. These are based on the idea that such very early stimulation can improve neural development, and perhaps prevent the normal massive nerve-cell death which usually takes place by the time babies are born (there is some evidence to support the latter). Animal studies have shown that prenatal-enrichment programmes can increase neural development in specific areas of the brain—for example, neuroanatomist Marion Diamond's research in California, in 1988, with baby rats. More importantly, studies on human babies, some small-scale but others with hundreds of subjects, have shown the same.

### THE PRENATAL CLASSROOM

Prenatal stimulation is not a new idea. It's an ancient traditional practice still observed tribally in Africa, Polynesia, and in urban Asia (where

Japanese mothers-to-be call it *taikyo*). However, the first of the new generation of prenatal learning programmes to reach the Western public was Californian obstetrician Dr. René Van de Carr's 1992 Prenatal Classroom. The work was subjected to the sort of scientific measurement in comparative studies which medical experts and well-informed members of the public understandably like to see before they give credence to any new idea.

The Prenatal Classroom system is used for five minutes twice daily. Parents are taught to reply to the first random kicks from the baby by patting the area where the kick landed, saying "Good baby! Kick again" (the "Kick Game"). According to

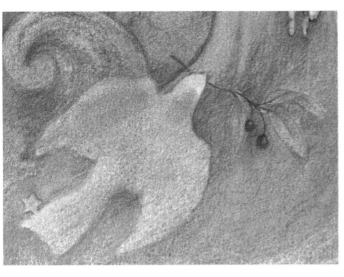

Dr. Van de Carr, the baby often learns to respond to this within a couple of weeks and starts kicking back. Other exercises involve pairing up words and actions—for example, the mother or father will say "stroke" several times, while stroking the area of the abdomen. The mothers are later taught more exercises, which involve

singing their babies songs, playing them musical scales on a xylophone, shining a torch on the area of their eyes to accustom them to the concept of light and dark, teaching them a list of 26 primary words and in the last month telling them stories. An extra plus of the programmes is that mothers report better pregnancies and births. It also appears that they are able to read their babies' needs and signals after the birth more easily than non-programme mothers.

Based on trials made in 1986 with 50 parents taking part fully, 50 part-timers and 50 not involved, researchers found the programme made differences in some areas. These were how mothers and fathers bonded with their babies; how early their babies began to talk; and whether mothers were able to breast-feed—which could arguably be at least partially explained by the parents' additional attention to, and involvement with, their babies, because of having to carry out the programme every day from the fifth month onward.

However, the researchers also found that the programme group of babies developed faster physically and that their milk teeth came through earlier, which cannot be explained by the extra attention from their parents. Another Dr. Van de Carr study of 20 babies and 20 controls also found that the experimental babies had higher Apgar scores (see p. 147) 5 minutes after birth.

But you don't need to study in a formal "classwomb" or structured programme, like Dr. Van de Carr's,

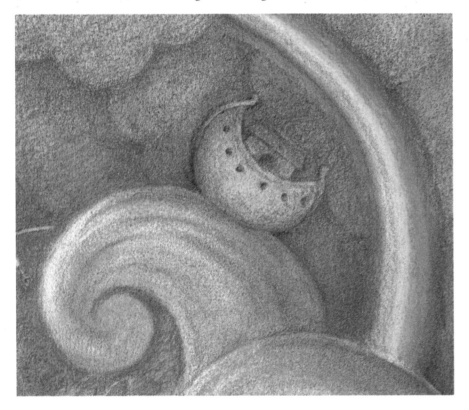

to start teaching your baby to respond to words from you—or your partner—while still in the womb. One couple, for example, found their baby already had excellent coordination and had learned to kick in a circle (see Games Your Unborn Baby Plays, p. 109).

### THE HUA CHIEW PROGRAMME

Some other positive benefits of the programmes which are hard to attribute to the extra attention from parents, were reported by another prenatal programme developed in Thailand in 1993. At the Hua Chiew Hospital, in Bangkok, the obstetrician Dr. Chairat Panthuraamphorn's system of prenatal stimulation began in the 12th week with a blissful ritual of relaxation, bathing, rocking in a chair, looking at beautiful pictures, listening to classical Thai music, abdominal massage, visualizing the baby and forthcoming birth, plus specific breathing exercises. At 20 weeks, the pregnant women also included in their programmes a daily 20-minute session involving tape recordings of their own voice and that of their partner, calling the baby's name, talking to him or her and playing light music. The programme goes on to include the music of bells, sounds from nature, fingertip massages, the "Kick Game" and spraying hot and cold water from a shower on the mother's abdomen to prepare the baby for the cooler temperatures outside the womb.

The Hua Chiew programme was tested using groups of 12 mothers carrying out the programme and 12 who did not. The experimental babies had significantly larger head circumferences and heights at two

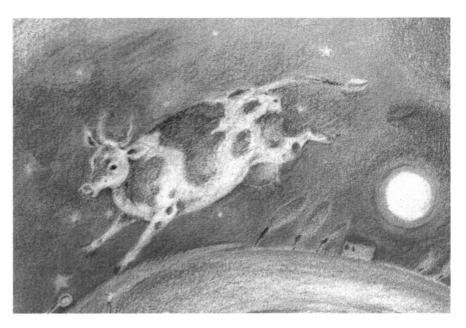

months, smiled in their first week, rolled over at one month, showed better motor-skill performance and speech development and learned new words more easily—also, when upset or angry, these babies could be calmed down faster than the controls, by rocking and patting.

### THE VENEZUELAN STUDY

The biggest study in this field, however, was led by psychologist Beatriz Manrique in Caracas, Venezuela, from 1990 to 1996, and involved 680 entire families. Pregnant women attended a 2-hour class for 13 weeks to learn how to communicate with their unborn babies. The results were assessed when the babies were two days, one month, eighteen months, and then three years old. The experimental babies had better hearing, language, memory, speech and motor skills. Researchers also found the mothers had been more confident and active during their labours, fared better with breastfeeding and showed more intense bonding with their babies. Also the

entire family appeared more stable. The Venezuelan government was so impressed it has decided to make the programme available nationwide.

### FIRSTART

One of the latest programmes under scientific scrutiny is called Firstart, from Valencia, Spain. Beginning at 28 weeks of pregnancy, the stimulation involves the sound of violins, which becomes progressively more complex as the unborn baby gets older. They are broadcast to the womb using a tape recorder, which the mother wears on a belt for up to 90 minutes a day. Parents are also encouraged to communicate with their unborn babies by talking to them, and to establish a loving relationship with them from before birth. In the first round of testing on a group of 101 Firstart babies six months after birth, babies had significantly more advanced skills, coordination and development than the babies who had not been part of the prenatal programme during the time inside their mothers.

# Sexuality During Pregnancy—What Your Baby May Notice

The effects of pregnancy on a couple's libido vary widely.
For the woman, a great deal depends on what stage of
pregnancy she is at and how well she is feeling.

The nausea and tiredness that affect most women (80 per cent) during their first three months of pregnancy are usually enough to put anyone off, but they generally fade by weeks 12 to 15. British obstetrician Dr. Adam Rodin, formerly of Guys & St. Thomas's Hospital, in London, estimates that about two-thirds of expectant mothers experience a surge of interest in lovemaking during the middle three months. Some even say they have never felt so sexual in their lives, nor been aroused so readily and easily. During the last two to three months, however, when a woman feels increasingly large and heavy, and perhaps has end-of-pregnancy tiredness creeping up on her, sexual interest tends to fade again.

Orgasms may also feel different for you—they can be more powerful, or your entire abdomen may harden, as it does during Braxton Hicks contractions (the painless practice contractions which are most noticeable towards the end of pregnancy). The 50 per cent increase in the amount of blood in the body can also result in some beneficial engorgement around the whole pelvic and vaginal area. This, and a huge increase in levels of sex hormones, may be partly why many women find they are more easily sexually aroused at this time. This pelvic-area engorgement can also make a woman's vagina feel "plumper". Her body's rapidly rising progesterone levels increase elasticity, as this hormone affects all the soft tissue (such as muscle) in the body.

### CONCERN FOR YOUR BABY

Lovemaking in later pregnancy is very unlikely to cause your labour to begin unless it is more or less ready to do so anyway. Nor is it going to harm your baby, who is protected by the plump, muscular ring of your cervix and the bag of amniotic fluid that surrounds it. Amniotic fluid is a good shock-absorber, especially while the baby has not yet begun to outgrow its environment and there is still plenty of room for liquid around it.

However, it is highly likely your baby will be aware of your lovemaking, especially if you—the mother—have an orgasm. This is partly because when you do so, your womb will contract, perhaps several times, as a normal reaction to the climax of pleasure. Although most top embryologists and obstetricians insist "your baby will notice nothing", Dr. David B. Chamberlain, President of the Association for Pre- and Perinatal Psychology and Health, says, "These doctors are 25 years behind the times. There have been at least two good studies showing the

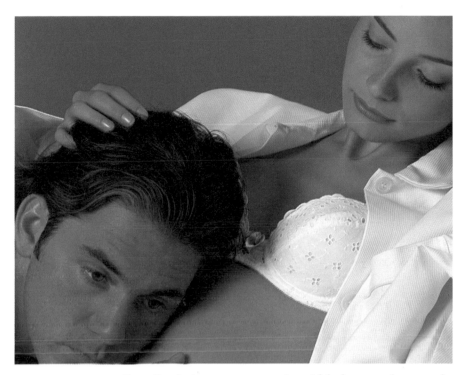

*ABOVE AND BELOW: Sexuality during pregnancy varies widely from couple to couple depending on the feelings of both the mother and the father.*

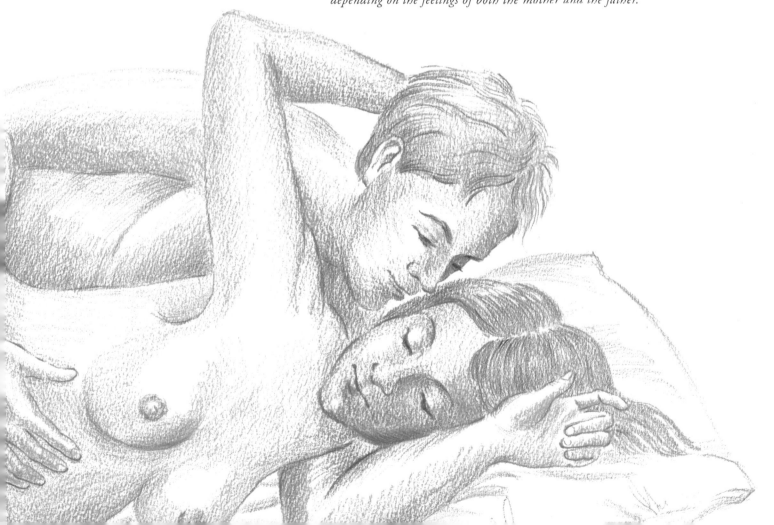

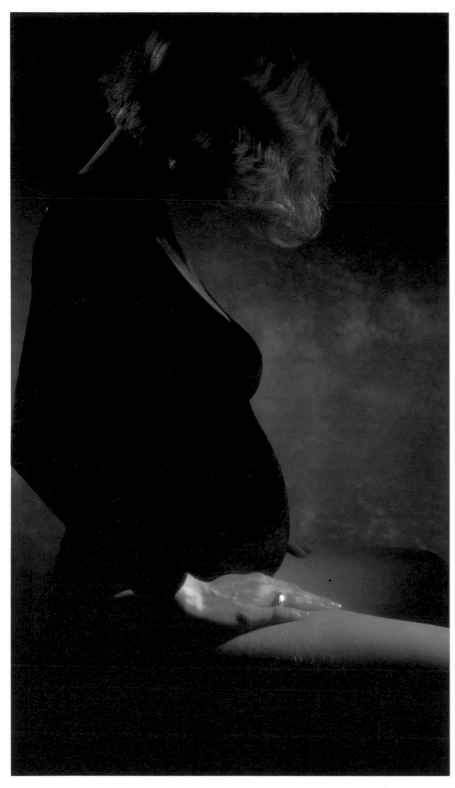

*ABOVE: Some women find their libido increases dramatically during pregnancy. Others may find that tiredness puts any ideas about making love out of their mind, at least for some of the time.*

opposite, and the reason there aren't more of these studies is they are very awkward to carry out. It's a very intimate thing for an expectant couple to do, wire themselves up in a laboratory situation and then make love."

One such piece of research was published in Scandinavia, in 1986, by Dr. Chayen, an American obstetrician who was only able to conduct the experiment because his work colleagues and their pregnant partners offered to help in the interests of science. Each couple was loaned monitors, which they were able to use in the privacy of their own homes.

The couples reported that when either the mother or the father reached an orgasm, it caused the foetus to become active in the womb, sometimes hyperactive; and after the father's climax, the foetus's heart rate sped up or slowed down by more than 30 beats a minute.

### WHAT YOUR BABY FEELS

However, it is thought that unborn babies are not able to bask directly in the benefits of intercourse's afterglow. According to embryologist Dr. Sammy Lee, "The natural opiate-like group of chemicals called endorphins, which the body makes after physical exercise—or lovemaking—that produce the feeling of euphoric relaxation are too large to cross the placental blood barrier and enter the foetus's own circulation". However, it is worth remembering that foetuses produce their own beta-endorphins as well.

That babies can and do share their mother's feelings is not just fanciful thinking, because there are dozens of research studies showing the direct effects of a mother's emotional state

## COMFORTABLE POSITIONS FOR MAKING LOVE DURING PREGNANCY ·

You don't have to start trying out new positions suddenly if you never liked the idea of them before. Making love during the later months of pregnancy is more a case of adapting what you both feel comfortable with to suit a woman's changing shape and an increased libido and sensitivity. Here are a few suggestions:

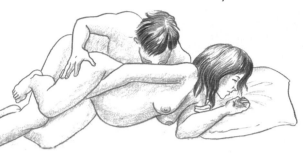

### SIDE-BY-SIDE

The man snuggles into his partner from behind. This is about as close as you can get towards the end of pregnancy when the bump of the growing baby will really come between you. This position does not put any pressure on a swelling abdomen, growing foetus or sensitive breasts.

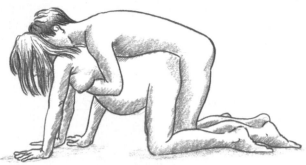

### FROM BEHIND

Kneeling on all fours, the male partner positions himself behind the woman. This does not create any pressure on her stomach or sensitive breasts. Also, this position makes it easier for a very pregnant woman to catch her breath if her belly is hanging downward (a possible problem in the last two to three months).

### MAN KNEELING

The woman sits on the edge of a bed or chair, while her partner kneels between her thighs. The height of the bed/chair is vital (you may have to try out a few options, so the man does not get cramp from having his knees partially bent). A variation if the abdomen is very large now is for the woman to lean back a bit on straight arms.

### WOMAN SITTING ASTRIDE

Again this position does not put any pressure on the woman's abdomen, and she can control the depth of penetration (her ripe cervix might be pressure-sensitive to strong thrusts of the penis). Some women feel self-conscious in this position ("I felt all he could see was this huge stomach and breasts") so prefer to wear a silky nightie or big, baggy T-shirt. Others feel both comfortable and sexually powerful when they are naked.

### INFANT SEXUALITY

Male foetuses have frequent erections inside the womb, and it is interesting that this often happens while they are sucking their thumbs. From a statistical point of view, according to research carried out in 1995 at Japan's Kyushu University in Fukuoka, in any 1 hour male babies aged 36 to 39 weeks have as many as 3 erections, each one lasting between 5 and 17 minutes. Apparently it is about the same for a newborn baby.

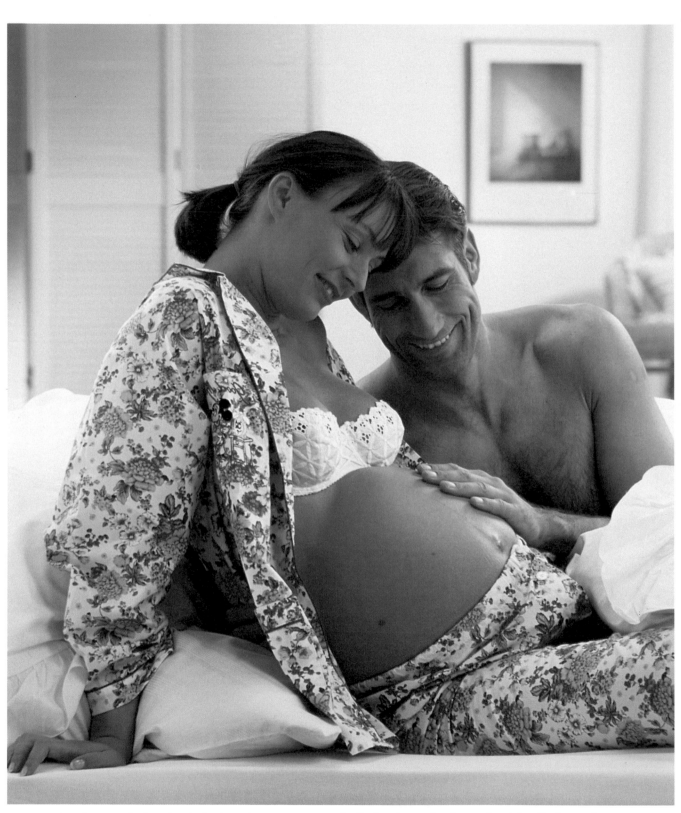

*ABOVE: A woman's changing body shape in pregnancy can be fascinating, seductive and exciting for her male partner, as the curves that epitomize femininity and fertility are exaggerated.*

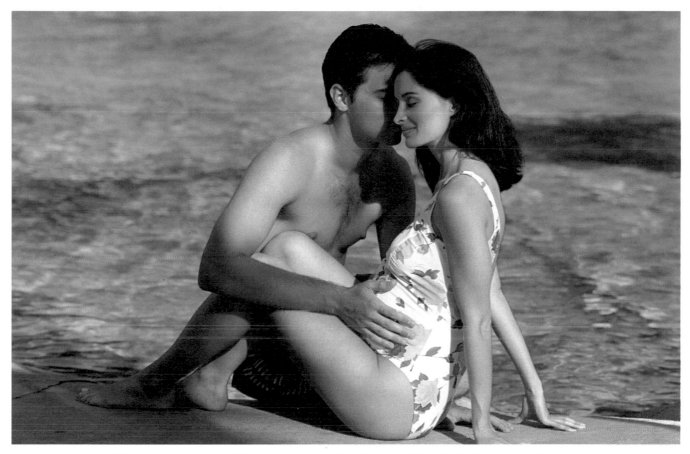

*ABOVE: Physical contact is good for all parties—mother, father and their baby. It can contribute to the sense of togetherness and the beginnings of feeling like a family.*

on the unborn (scc Docs Your Unborn Baby Feel Your Emotions?, p. 59). According to 1992 research on over 1,000 pregnant women by obstetrician Dr. Cheek, in San Francisco, California, there is also evidence of telepathy between mothers and their unborn babies.

### FATHERS AND SEXUALITY

Sometimes an expectant father will react powerfully to his partner's pregnancy, and to knowing there is a baby growing inside her, especially if he has been developing his own relationship with the unborn baby (perhaps talking to him or her, or stroking and patting his partner's abdomen). The many different feelings that expectant fathers mention are as individual as the men themselves. Just about all reactions are "normal", but they can affect a man's sexual attitude towards his partner.

Knowing a woman is carrying his child can be very exciting for some men, and many find the growing curves of pregnancy erotic, especially during the first four months, when the breasts are becoming so much fuller but body shape has not yet changed much in other ways. Others take the view that "I don't usually get excited by pregnant women, but because it's you and I helped to make you this shape, I still want to make love to you". Some feel it makes little difference; after all, the change is only temporary, and this is still the person they love. Others may feel, subconsciously, that being a mother has somehow put their partner in the category of "Mother"—someone who should be loved and respected, but not made love to.

A man can need some time to adjust to the idea of becoming a father, and to the fact that his partner is becoming a mother. If this is so, don't bottle up your emotions. Talk about the way you feel, and if you don't feel like making love, just enjoy kissing, hugging and caressing instead. This may sound like trite advice, because you have probably heard it many times before, but that does not make it any less true.

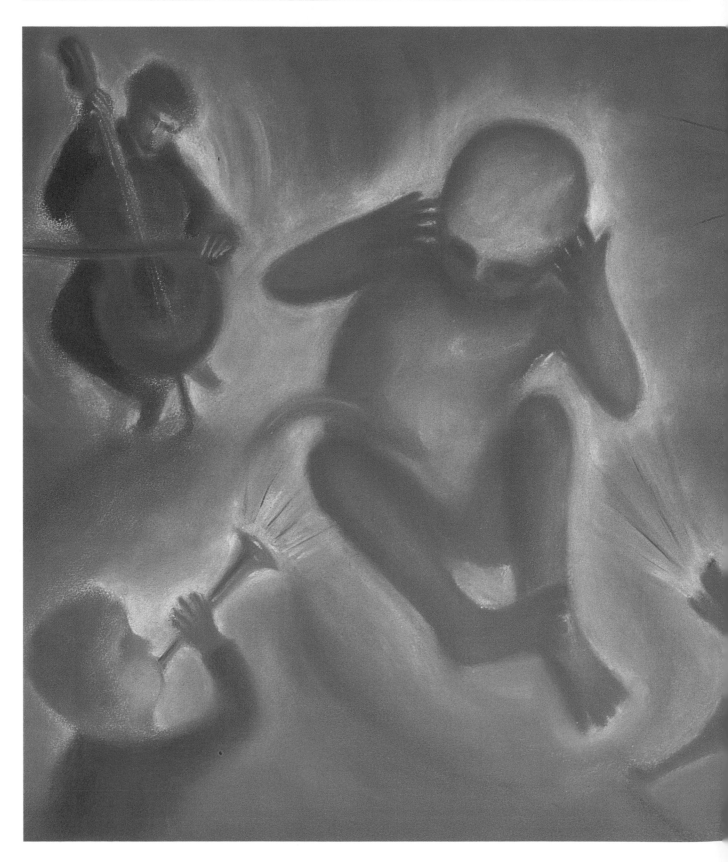

# What Your Baby Can Hear in the Womb

Of all the foetus's many different abilities and senses, hearing is the one scientists have studied the most because it is relatively easy to assess.

Since 1925, researchers have experimented with introducing foetuses to all sorts of different sounds, everything from music played through a loudspeaker, to door buzzers, fairy stories, soap opera theme-tunes and the whirr of an electric toothbrush.

Knowledge has come a long way, even in the past 25 years. As recently as the early 1970s, a textbook in paediatrics was teaching that newborn—let alone unborn—babies couldn't hear anything, despite the existence of research suggesting the opposite reaching as far back as 1925, when it was first reported that a foetus reacted powerfully to a car horn sounding nearby.

### HOW MUCH CAN BABIES REALLY HEAR?

Unborn babies start hearing as early as 12 weeks, according to Professor Peter Hepper, of Queen's University, in Belfast, Northern Ireland, and show their earliest response to sounds by a quickening or slowing heartbeat, or changes in the rate of eye blinking. As a rough guide, a foetus's heart rate will accelerate on hearing a loud sound, in a defensive reaction, but will slow down on hearing a softer sound, in what Columbia University's Pediatrics Department refers to as an "orienting or attention response".

Hepper's research shows babies did the latter—that is, became quiet, but attentive—when they heard the theme tune of of the Australian soap opera *Neighbours* after they were born, if their mothers had listened to it while they were pregnant. My own baby son, Ben, used to stop crying if it came on, even in the midst of a robust screaming fit. When he could crawl, he'd make for the television screen and stroke it with his fingers.

As to how much foetuses can hear most obstetricians would, even today, say "not much, apart from your own loud digestive gurglings and heartbeat, which can hit 85 decibels".

Again, science has proved them wrong. According to experiments conducted in 1989 with lambs still in the womb, French researchers at the University of Lille found that outside sounds reach the womb at the 30-decibel level—that's about half the loudness of a voice heard in an ordinary face-to-face conversation, which registers at between 65 and 70 decibels. The mother's voice is especially powerful because it is transmitted to her baby down through her body, so it reaches him or her more clearly than any outside sound.

Surgeon-turned-music-therapist Alfred Tomatis has his own research institute in Paris, where he trains the ears of expectant mothers and their babies for two hours a day with the music of Mozart. He likens a pregnant mother's body to a cello, explaining that it acts as a soundbox transmitting music (the mother's voice) to her baby in a series of vibrations, which stimulate the foetus's developing nervous system.

### REMEMBERING SOUNDS FROM THE WOMB

Babies also seem to remember what they have heard *in utero,* and many experiments have confirmed this. Your heartbeat is one of their favourites, and their memory of its

steady, comforting pulse and thud is probably why a baby finds it so reassuring being held close to your—or anyone else's—chest, or listening to the steady beat of a clock or clockwork wind-up toy. Cassette tapes (often expensive) of mothers' heartbeats and other womb sounds also appear to appeal to newborns, many of whom may find the relative quiet of their own cot and bedroom very disconcerting and not at all restful after inhabiting their mother's body all their life and being soothed by the sound effects her system continuously produced. Australian psychiatrist Dr. Albert Liley also believes the

familiarity of the mother's heartbeat from the time in the womb is the reason why most people prefer a metronome beat of 50 to 90 beats per minute above all others—because it's about the same range as a human heart. In addition, if pregnant women sing a specific lullaby or other tune, their babies prefer that one to any other after they are born. The same applies to phrases the foetuses heard regularly. They can even recognize stories, including, it seems, those read aloud to their pregnant mothers. One little boy insisted he'd heard *The Hobbit* before when his father first read it to him. And so he had, inside his mother, because her husband had read it to her when she was pregnant.

### HOW DO FOETUSES REACT TO SOUND?

Professor Hepper's work also shows that foetuses exhibit behavioural responses to sound by about 16 weeks. This idea is initially baffling because the ear is not even structurally complete until 24 weeks. However, perhaps it can be explained by the fact that, as some researchers suggest, an immature foetus is able to use the skin as a sense organ not just for touch, but also for registering sound, since there are receptors scattered across its surface for vibration as well as pain, temperature and touch. "This lends support to the idea that receptive hearing begins with the skin and the skeletal framework," suggests Dr. David B. Chamberlain, President of the Association for Pre- and Perinatal Psychology and Health, in the United States. Sound information from the vestibular and cochlear parts of the ear add to the early lis-

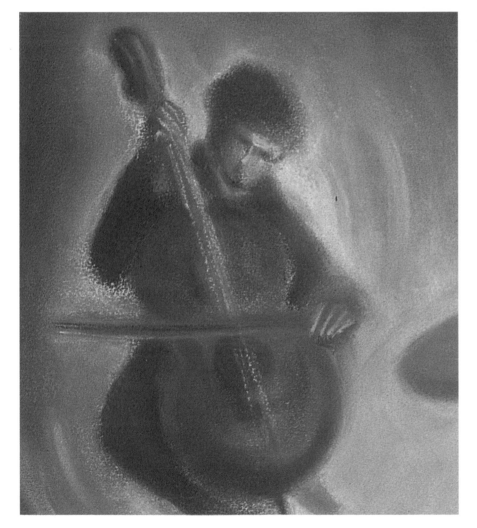

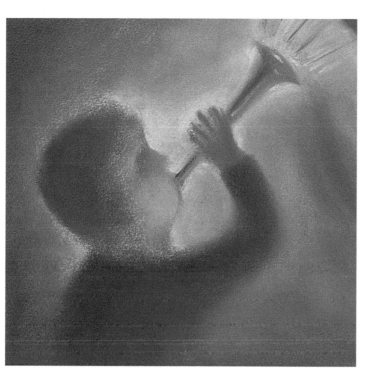

tening system as soon as these areas are sufficiently well developed to contribute.

## LANGUAGE LESSONS IN THE WOMB

High-tech analysis of premature babies' cries and their mothers' voices suggest foetuses develop intelligence very early. This enables them to learn the beginnings of speech from hearing your voice for up to six months in the womb.

Some doctors think this is absurd, believing you need language before you can be an intelligent being, but this idea leaves out something important—to learn a language, you have to be intelligent first to begin making sense of what you are hearing. The idea of babies taking language lessons in the womb was first suggested in 1975 by a Dr. Truby. Working with mothers and their (28-week-old) premature babies, he was the first person to use modern sound technology to analyse their voices. He found the rhythms of the babies' cries and intonations of the mothers' voices could be matched. The babies had absorbed and copied the very basic speech patterns of their mothers.

## UNDERSTANDING WHAT YOU SAY

Most mothers talk to the babies growing in their womb, either in their heads or aloud, and are often laughed at good-naturedly for doing so ("They can't understand you, don't be silly"). Can't they just?

Any corporate communications expert will tell you there are two levels to successful communication, and what someone actually says out loud in words is only the first of those levels. The second is the sub-text— what it is you sense the other person means, or even just the unspoken message conveyed which is never said aloud. It appears, then, that mothers and their unborn babies use both these conversational or dialogue skills interchangeably.

After working with 1,000 subjects in 1992, San Franciscan obstetrician David Cheek made a plausible case for the existence of everyday telepathy between mothers and their unborn babies. In 1995, a team of obstetricians in Phoenix, Arizona, used an electronically synthesized voice to "talk" babies out of difficult breech positions, which usually require Caesarean delivery, and getting them to turn around. This suggests that babies understand what you say to

them, either silently or in words out loud.

Nurses and midwives have reported the same reaction from babies using normal but very emphatic forms of human speech. None of these things would be happening if our messages to the unborn child were not being received, and at least partially understood.

Perhaps this is not as odd as it may sound. Adult couples who are emotionally very close often pick up on each others' thoughts and feelings without verbal cues, as do mothers with small children. Another possible example of mother-baby telepathic communication is the way a breast-feeding mother will, time and again, wake seconds or minutes before her baby does at night, even if he or she is not in the same room.

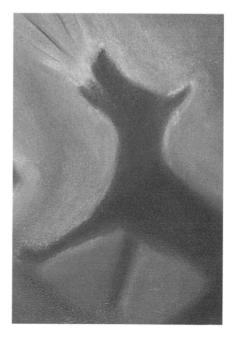

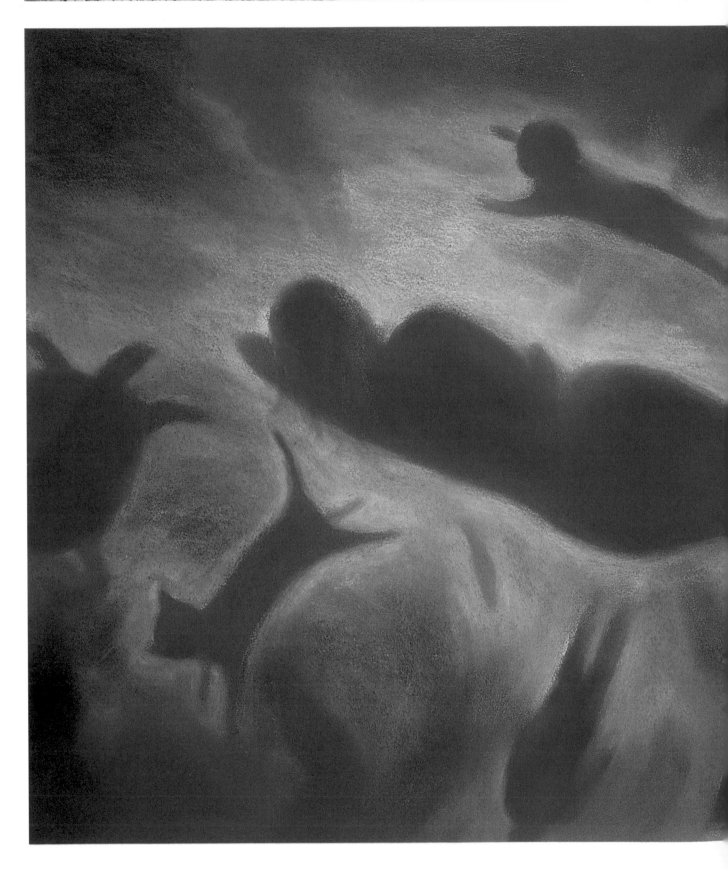

# The Dreams of Pregnant Women and Their Unborn Babies

**Mothers-to-be often report having vivid and haunting dreams during their pregnancies.**

The dreams of pregnancy may be blissful, serene, calming, exciting, joyous, disquieting, puzzling or even downright alarming. Suddenly having such dreams can be quite disconcerting if you have never been especially aware of any before, or have merely registered you had some sort of vague dreams but could never remember anything much about them when you woke up.

However, having powerful dreams in pregnancy is considered normal and healthy by many psychologists, including Dr. Thomas Verny, regarded by many people as the founding father of popular prenatal psychology in the United States. Apparently many of the dreams of pregnant women can be interpreted as expressing their unconscious feelings—often mixed—about their unborn baby or the impending birth. These dreams can, therefore, have beneficial effects. According to Dr. Verny, the advantages vary from feeling more "sorted out" about the idea of a baby, especially if it is your first, to solidly practical benefits, such as shorter labours and easier childbirths.

## COMMON THEMES

In 1995, Eileen Stukane, author of *The Dream Worlds of Pregnancy*, interviewed several hundred pregnant women about their nocturnal imaginings, and found they shared many common characteristics. During the first three months the recurring images seemed to be fertile and soothing—cats, birds, sheep, flowers, lambs and other young animals and water in the form of seas, rivers and lakes. These are thought to represent the awareness that you are a fertile woman, but also the difficulty most newly pregnant women have trying to imagine a small embryo or foetus inside them when there is, as yet, so little to show for it on the outside.

## WORRIES REVEALED

Around the fourth month, Stukane reported many women started to have more worrying dreams: being marooned or stuck up trees were common subjects at this time, suggesting feelings of isolation, a certain helplessness and a mildly panicky sense of "well this is it. I'm committed to having the baby now". As the subjects' bellies swelled and they felt increasingly bulky and cumbersome, cars, lorries and houses all became common dream subjects. Finally, as the birth approached, many women dreamed of trying to look at or meet their future son or daughter. My own interviewees mentioned dreaming of unzipping the womb wall and rezipping it; of having see-through

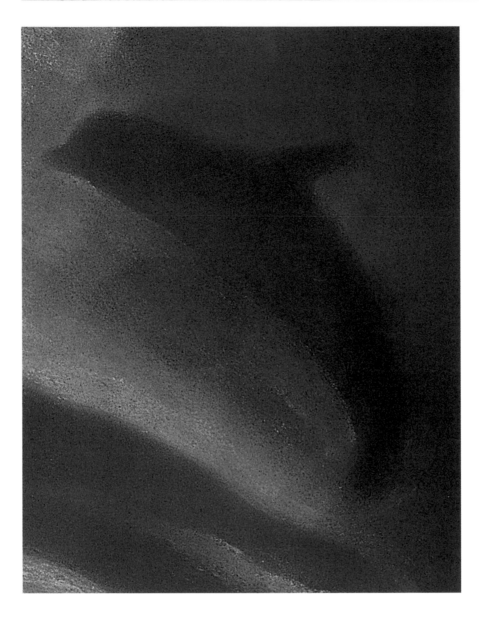

of memory track begin streaking across the foetal brain" during the final three months. Sonographic research conducted in the early 1980s in the United States and reported in the *American Journal of Roentology* shows rapid eye-movement (REM) sleep, which indicates dreaming, can be detected at about 23 weeks, before 7 months. That potentially gives babies 17 weeks to dream in the womb before birth.

REM sleep encourages a foetus's brain to develop, which may be why it spends about 60 per cent of its last 3 months in the womb in this state. Newborns dream for about 8 hours a day, although the amount of time gradually diminishes with age: younger adults spend about 20 per cent of their sleep time in REM. However, this may not just be because dreaming is something a foetus does as it becomes more like an adult approaching its birth. According to research conducted in the early 1990s in Japan, the opposite is true: it is more likely that when children and adults sleep and dream, it is actually *they* who are reverting back to their original in-the-womb mental state.

### WHAT YOUR BABY DREAMS ABOUT

You may think there is little for a foetus to dream about. Don't adults use dreaming as a means of unravelling the thousands of worries and impressions of their day? What, then, are babies doing that is so thought-provoking? Plenty that they find interesting enough to relive while asleep, says Dr. Verny, who argues that foetuses dream about the things they have been doing too— moving their feet and hands, playing

womb walls "a bit cloudy", and of trying to peer through misted-up windows at what they knew was their baby's face on the other side. By examining the content of the dreams themselves, and the way they make you feel when you wake up, you can confront, talk about, and often deal with many of the concerns you have about being pregnant, the coming birth itself or the child whose mother you will soon become.

### YOUR BABY DREAMS TOO

It's not just your own sleeping imagination that's running riot, though. Your baby is dreaming right along with you for much of your pregnancy. He or she cannot help sensing your more powerful thoughts and feelings (see Does Your Unborn Baby Feel Your Emotions?, p. 59) because you are sharing a body in both a physical and psychological sense. According to Dr. Verny, "the first thin slivers

with the umbilical cord, hearing sounds, and reliving any powerful emotions the mother may have experienced that day and of which they have also been aware, for example, blissful peace through to alarm, delight, irritation or stress.

Newborn babies (up to a week or so old) give us an additional clue as to how unborn babies dream *in utero* as their neurological development is very similar to a baby at, say, 36 weeks' gestation. Their dreaming faces register puzzlement, fright and even disdain. As their expressions change, they also make some accompanying writhing movements with their body and limbs, or curl, clench and splay their fingers and toes, just as you might expect someone who was having a powerful dream to behave.

Observers in the 1960s also reported smiles and expressions of amusement on the faces of newborns and babies only a few days old, even though most paediatricians insist it's "just wind" and that new babies cannot smile until they are six weeks old. Perhaps social smiles in response to a smile from a parent are the type which begin at six weeks, but what psychologists call cognitive smiles (that is, coming from within, from the baby's own feelings) can sometimes be seen from day one while the baby sleeps.

This is all part of the growing body of evidence suggesting that unborn babies are indeed (as argued in 1994 by Dr. David B. Chamberlain, President of the Association for Pre- and Perinatal Psychology and Health) "processing

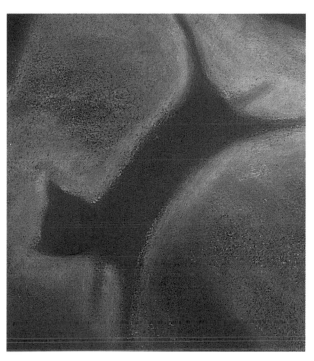

their own thoughts, feelings and life experiences to date, much as the rest of us do in dreams".

## DO BABIES SHARE YOUR DREAMS?

Does your unborn baby ever sense your dreams (especially if they are very powerful, frightening or soothing) in the same way as they can pick up on your moods (see Does Your Unborn Baby Feel Your Emotions,

p. 59)? There is evidence that mothers and their unborn babies use several different forms of wordless communication via the hormonal route—down the umbilical cord's blood supply—and the psychic route.

No one knows if intense dreams travel the same routes, but it is interesting to note that the indigenous people of the southern highlands of New Guinea act out the possibility on a regular basis. This they call "Dream Inducement" and entire communities take part, as a mystery- or problem-solving exercise. For instance, if someone dies from suspected witchcraft, the villagers join together in "seeker-dreaming" to find out who did it. Sleeping together with ropes connecting their wrists and chests (a symbolic umbilical cord?), a "Dream Master" watches over them, and coordinates the clues they dream of. It is believed that when two people dream the same thing the dream has travelled along the cords that join them, as in a telephone cable.

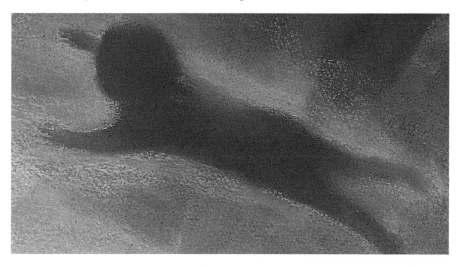

# Twins and You

## One in 85 mothers now gives birth to twins, or has multiple births, compared to 1 in a 100, 15 years ago.

More mothers are having multiple births, perhaps because more couples are having fertility treatment, often with ovulation-stimulating drugs and/or the IVF implantation of up to four or five embryos.

If you are carrying twins, they may be fraternal (that is, have developed from two different eggs fertilized by two separate sperm). They will be no more alike than any other brothers or sisters. But if your twins are the result of a single egg fertilized by one sperm, which split in half at a very early stage and developed from there, your babies will be identical twins. About one in every three pairs of twins is identical. With fraternal twins, roughly half are one boy and one girl, with the rest equally divided between dissimilar girl pairs and dissimilar boy pairs.

### COPING WITH A TWIN PREGNANCY

A mother pregnant with twins may sail through her pregnancy, and there isn't any medical reason why she shouldn't. However, carrying two (or three, or four...) babies inside you is harder work for your body. You are likely to put on weight faster than if you are carrying a single baby, and to put on more weight overall because you have two (or more) babies, placentas and often amniotic sacs and volumes of amniotic fluid—in fact, your total pregnancy gain can be up to half your usual weight. You may also experience pregnancy discomforts such as tiredness and nausea more acutely than other women, and feel very heavy in the last few weeks. But you are also more likely to have a shorter pregnancy: the average is 35 to 37 weeks instead of 40, and your babies may be lighter, at around 2.5 kg ($5^{1}/_{2}$ pounds) each, rather than 3.15 kg (7 pounds).

You may need Caesarean delivery, as it is not easy for both twins to be in the right position (head down) to be born. As they are likely to be smaller if they arrive before 37 weeks (technically, premature), and if they have had a less-than-easy birth, one or both twins might need to be put under observation in a special-care baby unit for a short while.

Your obstetrician and/or midwife will probably monitor your pregnancy quite closely, because there are sometimes certain problems associated with multiple pregnancies, although good antenatal care should mean they are spotted early, and treated effectively. These can include: high blood pressure; pre-eclampsia; one baby growing more slowly than the other; and one of the babies lying breech (bottom first) or transverse (across the womb). The most usual positions are either both vertex, meaning head down (which is fine), for about half of all twin pairs; or top to tail, in which case your obstetrician may be able to turn one around. If he or she cannot, you will probably be advised to have your babies by Caesarean section. Other potential problems are loss of one of the foetuses in a miscarriage, although the other continues healthily to term; and early re-absorption of one of the embryos ("Vanishing Twin Syndrome").

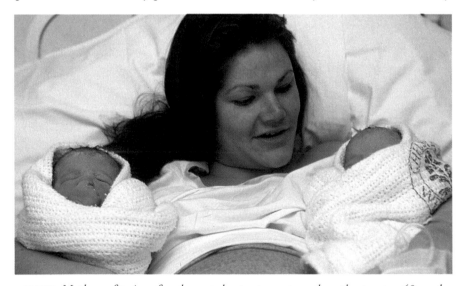

*ABOVE: Mothers of twins often have a shorter pregnancy than the average 40 weeks, but they are likely to put on more weight.*

*ABOVE: Twins are almost always either both awake, or both asleep, at the same time. They often find each other a hugely reassuring, comforting presence and parents frequently realize that they will not sleep or settle if they are not together.*

### TWINS IN THE WOMB

There is a small, but growing, body of research suggesting that to develop with your twin alongside you in your mother's womb is a very special experience, one which nurtures a depth of understanding, comfort and intimacy that non-twins can only guess at.

If a twin dies in the womb, leaving the other alone (Vanishing Twin Syndrome), this can profoundly affect the lone survivor, says paediatrician Elizabeth Bryan, of Queen Charlotte's Hospital, in London, who specializes in multiple births.

She adds that some lone twins have personality problems which appear to be related to the loss of their brother or sister, and twins whose sibling was stillborn seem to be especially profoundly affected. "If one dies, the other [twin] surely knows it," according to Dr. David B. Chamberlain, President of the Association for Pre- and Perinatal Psychology and Health. "The effect is very variable, but the symptoms later in life are those of loneliness, abandonment and grief. They are sad about something they cannot put a name to—and they are often

unconsciously looking for their twin." (See Memories of Being in the Womb—and Being Born, p. 121.) Estimates as to how often this happens vary from 4 per cent to 10 per cent of cases.

The positive side of the special relationship between twins is that they can be immensely sensitive to each other's needs, mutually consoling and emotionally close, both *in utero* and outside. Studies suggest that twin babies can calm each other from a very young age—at five or six months they will even routinely suck each other's thumbs—and when left

## DEVELOPMENT AND POSITIONING OF TWINS

Twins can be identical or non-identical depending on their route of development, illustrated below.

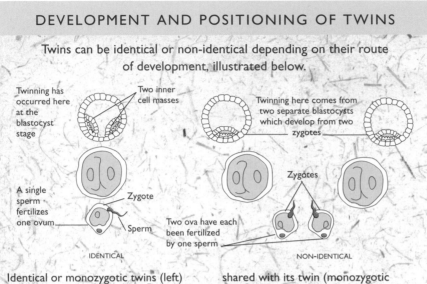

Twinning has occurred here at the blastocyst stage

Two inner cell masses

Twinning here comes from two separate blastocysts which develop from two zygotes

A single sperm fertilizes one ovum

Zygote

Sperm

Two ova have each been fertilized by one sperm

Zygotes

IDENTICAL

NON-IDENTICAL

Identical or monozygotic twins (left) grow from *one single* egg, fertilized by *one single* sperm, which grows into a single cell bundle containing not one but two, separate embryos. Each one develops into a baby with its own umbilical cord and (usually) its own amniotic sac—but having to draw its food and oxygen from one placenta

shared with its twin (monozygotic twinning at the two-cell stage results in each of the twins having its own placenta). Non-identical twins (right) develop when two separate egg cells are fertilized by two separate sperm, and each grows into a separate embryo, with its own placenta. They are no more alike than any other brothers or sisters.

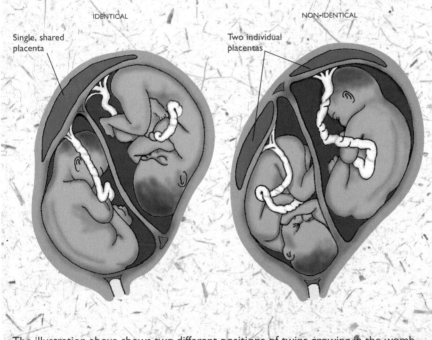

IDENTICAL

NON-IDENTICAL

Single, shared placenta

Two individual placentas

The illustration above shows two different positions of twins growing in the womb. Those on the left share a placenta and are identical, monozygotic twins. Each of the pair on the right has its own placenta. They are probably fraternal, non-identical twins, although they may be monozygotic twins which formed at the two-cell stage.

together they remain content for longer periods of time than single babies do, each soothed by the presence of the other. Parents of twins from the British Twins and Multiple Births Association note these babies often sleep best in cots flush next to each other, and if moved will begin repeated night-waking.

### TWINS OUTSIDE THE WOMB

There is some evidence to suggest this closeness begins while the babies are developing inside their mothers, and any behavioural patterns and relationships which start in the womb continue after the babies are born, into childhood, and often throughout adulthood, too. In the early 1990s, child psychoanalyst Dr. Alessandra Piontelli, in Milan, used ultrasound imaging to compare babies' lives in the womb with the way they behaved afterwards. She watched eight twin pregnancies at monthly intervals from the 18th week, and then recorded the children throughout infancy and early childhood. She noted that one pair of twin girls, Marisa and Beatrice, kicked each other repeatedly while inside their mother, and as infants and small children continued doing so. In her book, *From Foetus to Child*, she describes another pair, one dominant, the other submissive. When the dominant twin pushed or hit him, the other withdrew and laid his head on the cushion of the placenta, apparently retreating there. When they were four years old, they still had a similar relationship: if there was tension or fighting, the more passive twin would put his head upon a special pillow which he often carried with him to use as his security blanket.

Yet another pair behaved very differently. At 20 weeks, Luca was very active, kicking and changing positions constantly, but periodically he would turn his attention to his quieter, sleepier sister, waking her by reaching out with his hands to touch her face through the amniotic membrane dividing them, while she responded by turning her face towards him. They would rub cheeks, appear to kiss and hug, stroke each other's faces and rub their feet together before going back to their original, separate activities. At the age of one, a favourite game played by the twins was to sit on different sides of a curtain, with Luca, just as he used to do in the womb, putting out his hand to touch Alicia's head. She still responded by inclining her head towards him, except this time their contact was accompanied by smiles and gurgles.

Such records are rare, but there are others—for example, researcher Brigit Arabin's video of twins kissing *in utero*, with the receiving twin wearing what Arabin describes as a blissful expression.

There have also been strict clinical trials charting synchronicity in twins. One was carried out in 1992 at Baltimore's Johns Hopkins University School of Medicine, where researchers monitored two physiological functions—heart beat and foetal movement. In a third of cases they found that if one foetus's heart rate accelerated or slowed, the other twin's would do so, too, at exactly the same time. They also found that nearly half of the twins' periods of moving about perfectly coincided with each other, and that they were almost always (94.7 per cent of the time) either awake or asleep at the same time.

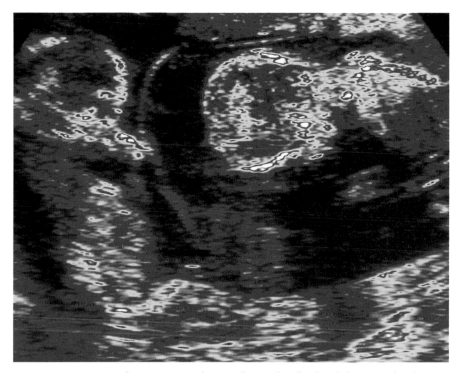

*ABOVE: Twins caught on scan in the womb: one has his head down and is lying horizontally, one is sitting upright. Both are in separate amniotic sacs (the dark areas). Later they will settle into more space-saving positions (see p.106).*

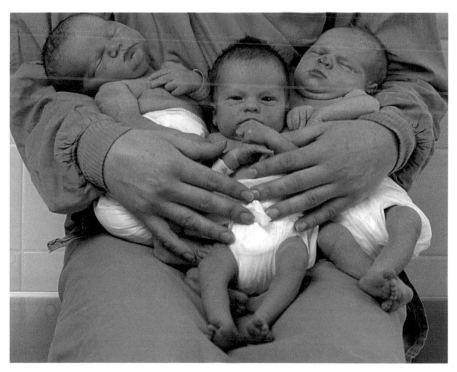

*ABOVE: As the use of assisted fertilization treatments by couples increases, triplets and other multiple births are becoming much more common than they were even 20 years ago.*

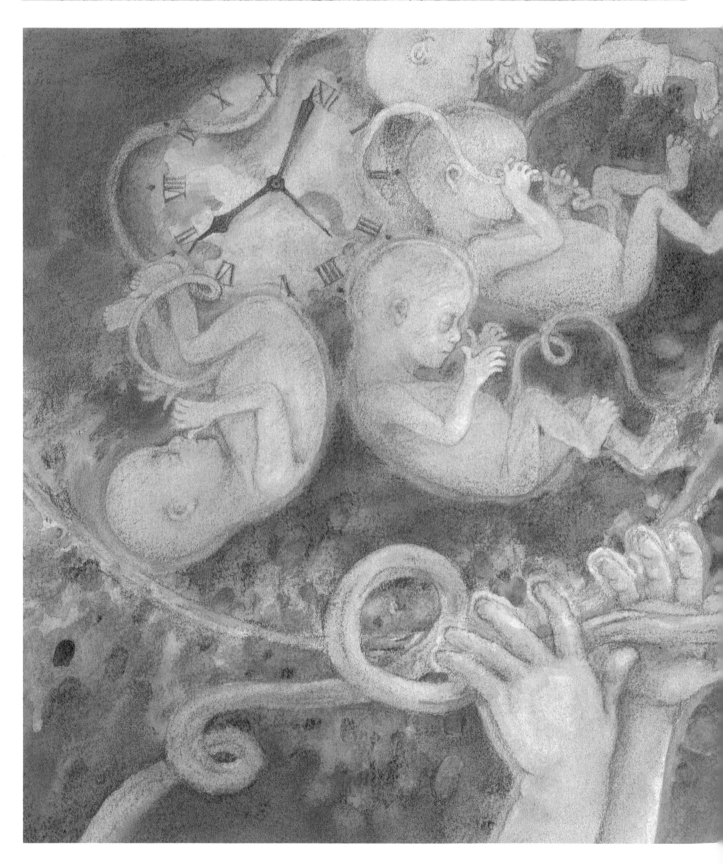

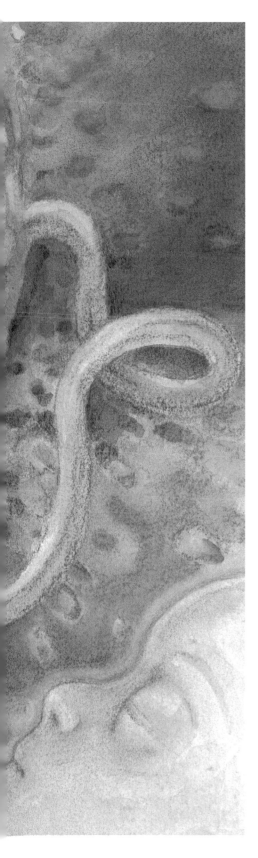

# Games Your Unborn Baby Plays

**Parents can teach their unborn babies to play games with them even while they are still developing in the womb.**

Unborn babies often play "games" by themselves, or, if they are part of a set of twins, they play with their brother or sister, setting the tone for the way they will interact together and the roles they take with each other after they are born.

One Canadian father used to come home at the same time each evening from work, and in fun called "hoo, hoo!" next to his partner's swelling abdomen. But he realized after a while that his child would be ready and waiting for him, as one night around the 25th week of pregnancy, a small foot kicked out into his cheek on whatever side he spoke on. Father and baby continued to play this game together until birth.

### THE "KICK GAME"

From about 20 weeks' gestation, foetuses can be taught to play the "Kick Game", according to Dr. Rene Van de Carr, the Californian obstetrician whose Prenatal Classroom Program (see What Your Unborn Baby Can Learn, p. 87) has thousands of infant graduates. Babies learn to kick back in response to the mother pressing or patting her own abdomen, while saying "kick, kick!" Or, when then the baby kicks, the mother responds with "There's a good baby!" This is not only meant to stimulate neurologically, it can be the first real communication between you and your unborn baby.

There is nothing to stop fathers or siblings from pressing, patting or speaking to babies in the womb, either, most effectively through a hollow cardboard tube. Mothers won't need that, because their voice reverberates down through the body, reaching the baby surprisingly well.

### THE UMBILICAL CORD— NOT JUST A FOOD SUPPLY

Foetuses also play with their umbilical cords, their lifelines, bringing vital food and oxygen dissolved in the mother's own blood supply. The cord is also a major "consoling presence", as researcher and hypnotherapist Mary Straub puts it. A foetus will grip its own umbilical cord experimentally and "this may be a source of real comfort and embryonic pleasure," according to Straub. By the time babies reach six months, the size of the hand and the circumference of the cord are relatively proportional, and their grip can be a very strong one—premature infants can support their own weight by holding on to a person's fingers (although they lose this ability about two months after birth). Straub suggests unborn babies can clutch their own umbilical cords hard enough to cause the partial stoppage of their own oxygen supply, which "mimics the psychological effects of high emotion". In fact, this may give the foetus a self-administered adrenaline rush of excitement.

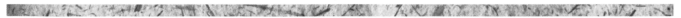

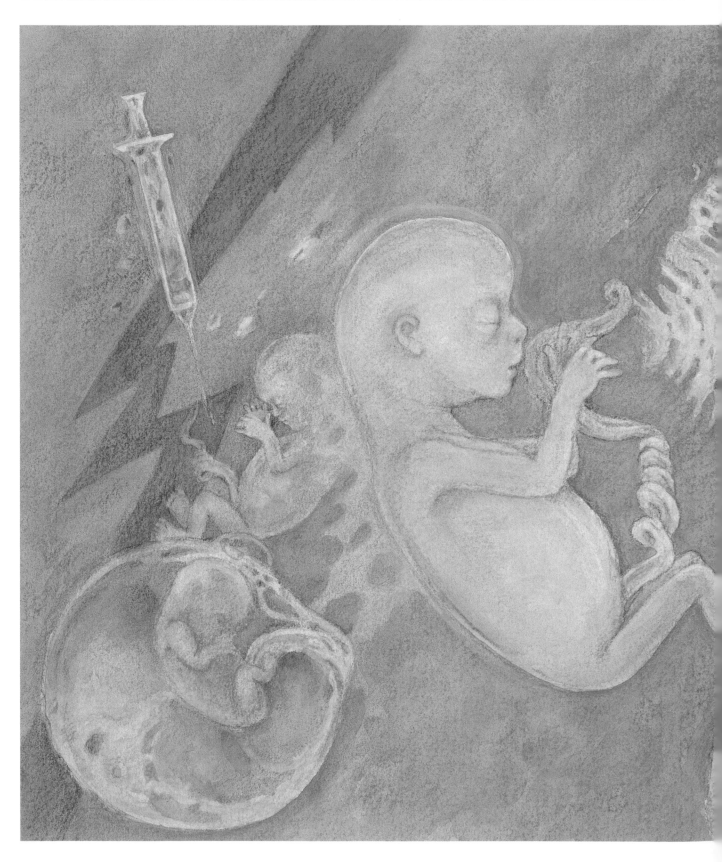

# Can Preborns and Newborns Feel Pain?

## Foetal sentience awareness is of enormous importance: if preborn and unborn babies do indeed experience pain, what can we do to help?

The question of whether babies are capable of feeling pain or discomfort during birth, as soon as they are born or even before they are born, is not only extremely important, but also loaded emotionally, ethically and scientifically. And like all really important, but uncomfortable, issues, it is not going to go away.

This is partly because the birth of each new baby usually raises this question in the minds of at least some of those involved, usually the parents ("Did the forceps hurt? Was that scalp monitor uncomfortable?"), and partly because, for better or worse, the question of whether the preborn or just-born baby feels pain, is, thanks to new research, becoming highly topical. It involves high-profile arguments, powerful gut reactions and heated scientific debates, all aired in public via the medical and consumer media, drawing a wide range of reactions from groups as diverse as parents, philosophy lecturers, anti-abortion groups, obstetricians, nurses, midwives, medical ethics experts, psychiatrists, psychotherapists and politicians.

### THE NEED FOR RESEARCH

The issue of what foetuses and newborns feel has to be confronted and dealt with because, like the entire field of foetal sentience (awareness), it has enormous and far-reaching implications. Many of these are potentially very positive, others are deeply worrisome. Most people's immediate and natural reactions seem compounded equally of pity, alarm, denial and guilt, but none of these is going to be of any help in practical terms to the unborn or newborn babies.

What *will* help is well-researched, worldwide agreement between all the different branches of the medical profession—many of whom do not usually discuss issues together at all—in the fields of foetal medicine and obstetrics.

Unborn babies and their parents would also benefit greatly from the setting up of a standardized, internationally recognized and properly implemented system of measures to guarantee when a foetus or newborn is capable of feeling pain or discomfort, since all medical practitioners are obliged to cause as little as possible. This applies whether a baby is undergoing vital surgery in the womb, being medically aborted, having difficulties coming down the birth canal, experiencing assisted delivery with forceps or ventouse or being monitored with a scalp electrode. It also covers premature babies being looked after in special-care baby units, and even healthy, full-term babies who are being taken from their mother immediately after birth to be weighed, measured, and to have their reflexes briskly checked for standard Apgar scoring (see p. 147).

### SCHOOLS OF THOUGHT

There are three main schools of thought with regard to the issue of pain in unborn and newborn babies.

The first is that foetuses and newborns do not feel pain like we do. Many doctors argue that you can only feel pain if you have experienced it before and remember the context in which it happened. They claim, therefore, that foetuses—and some experts still say this goes for newborns, too—only show automatic reflex actions to painful stimuli, and to them it is not actually painful "as such".

The two pieces of research that did most to establish this idea were carried out in 1925 at Northwestern University, in Chicago, and Chicago's Lying-In Hospital, and in 1941 at Columbia University and The Babies' Hospital, in New York. The former tests involved researchers poking pins into newborn babies' cheeks, thighs and calves. Although virtually all reacted in the first hours and first day after birth, it was noted that their reactions became sharper from days 1 to 12. The researchers concluded that newborns were not very sensitive at birth but that they became progressively more so. Unfortunately, the hospitals had failed to take into account the fact that all the mothers had had anaesthetic drugs during labour and delivery, and that these had therefore entered the babies' systems as well, temporarily dulling their reactions to pain.

The latter research also tested newborns' sensitivity using pin-pricks. The doctors recorded "diffuse bodily movements accompanied by crying and possibly a local reflex" when pins were stuck into the babies. Their use of the term "reflex" indicated that they thought there could not be a mental or emotional component in their reactions to pain, because their brains were not yet sufficiently developed.

Because of this type of thinking, many newborn baby boys, even today, still have their penises circum-

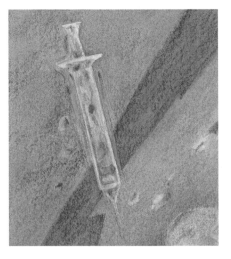

cised without pain relief; also, up until about the mid-1980s, newborns were having emergency operations without anaesthetic. It was believed that not only were the babies' systems too immature for them to feel pain "as such", but also that the side effects of anaesthesia could be damaging. Understandably, the death rate of these babies was high, usually from sheer shock. In 1986, two American parents mounted a major pressure campaign, both about this and about the fact that premature babies, and in some cases infants up to 15 months old, had no anaesthetics for their operations either. The practice was changed.

A second view is that foetuses can experience pain in the womb from about 9 weeks. It is argued that enough of the foetus's rudimentary neurological system has developed by then, and that even though the cerebral cortex has not yet formed, the lower centres of the brain, such as the brainstem, can carry out some of the cortex's functions.

Much has been made of this (such as the "Foetal Sentience Report", published by an anti-abortion coalition in the United Kingdom in 1996) as an argument against termination except at very early stages.

Yet another view holds that it is probable that the older foetus feels pain. "It is unlikely to do so under 13 weeks, and between 13 and 26 weeks, we don't know… We should, therefore, err on the safe side and treat the foetus as if it does feel pain, even though it may not," explains Dr. Vivette Glover, foetal sentience expert and clinical scientist at Queen Charlotte's Hospital, in London. The paediatrics unit based at Queen Charlotte's, under Professor Nicholas Fisk, is consequently working on giving the opiate drug fentanyl to foetuses who need life-saving transfusions.

### BABIES' SEMAPHORE

"Do newborns feel pain? Of course. There are many objective signs if you believe what you observe," says Dr. David B. Chamberlain. A straightforward checklist of the standard indicators of pain in a person of any age can be offered as evidence.

### Crying

Spectrographs showing changes in pitch and pattern reflect just how much or how little something hurts.

Listen to the cries of just-born babies—often they are powerful, outraged and alarmed. In 1986, research recording newborn babies' cries during circumcision without anaesthetic precisely reflected the degree of invasiveness of the surgery.

### Facial Expressions

A creased or furrowed brow, quivering chin and lips, wide open mouth and pursed lips all communicate distress or pain in any age-group.

### Body Movements

A baby's response to painful stimuli is to jerk away, pull back, swing its arms, push with its hands and frantically chafe one leg against the other.

### Breathing and/or Heart Rate Changes

Newborn babies' heart rates can shoot up by 50 beats per minute (bpm), to 180 bpm in response to pain. Heart response to pain can also be measured in foetuses.

Yet other indicators are used to guage whether pain or discomfort is being registered in foetuses.

### Stress Hormones

Hormones, such as cortisol, are released by foetuses, infants and adults in response to stress or pain—when someone is in pain his or her levels may rise threefold or fourfold. In 1995, a team comprising five surgeons led by Professor Xenophon Giannakoulopoulos, at Queen Charlotte's Hospital, in London, found that during foetal blood transfusions via the liver, the unborn babies' blood levels of cortisol nearly doubled, and their endorphin (natural painkiller) output increased by 600 per cent. This is regarded as the first piece of conclusive proof that unborn babies

can feel pain, fear and stress. Professor Nicholas Fisk, who was part of the research team, is currently working with a unit on the island of Jersey to see what the babies' stress hormone responses are to forceps and vacuum delivery.

### Memories

Under hypnosis, children's or adults' memories of both prenatal and birth trauma can be vivid and remarkably accurate. These include recall of

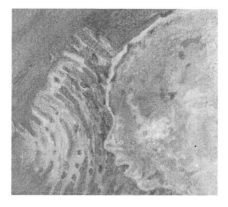

painful labour/birth procedures and events (see Memories of Being in the Womb—and Being Born, p. 121).

### WHAT CAN WE DO ABOUT IT?

If you feel, as many people now do, that a baby can experience discomfort and/or pain during birth, you can help your own considerably.

First, don't give permission for surgery on your baby, including circumcision, without firm assurance that adequate painkilling anaesthesia will be used.

Secondly, tell your doctor what procedures you want to avoid, and find alternatives for painful procedures or postpone them for as long as possible after the baby's birth. This is because the earliest experiences of pain may be the most upset-

ting and may produce the deepest memory imprint.

Thirdly, learn and use drug-free pain-relief measures to help make your labour more comfortable and the delivery calmer and more relaxed (and, therefore, more comfortable) for your baby.

The list of self-help measures is long, and features, very encouragingly, many things you may be already planning to use anyway. These include: relaxation techniques, such as breathing and visualization, autogenic training or self-hypnosis; and complementary therapies, such as homoeopathy, reflexology, acupressure and aromatherapy, to support the birth process and reduce any pain you may experience; labouring/giving birth in water; moving about freely; trying to remain in upright—squatting, sitting, leaning or kneeling—positions rather than lying flat on your back; talking to and reassuring your baby either out loud or in your head (it seems they can hear you—see p. 99 on research on telepathy between mothers and their unborn babies); having a supportive companion—your partner, a friend, relative, a trusted nurse, midwife or doctor—with you; trying to avoid obstetric interventions, such as the rupture of the amniotic sac membranes or forceps delivery unless necessary; trying to avoid a labour induced by oxytocin drip, the powerful, abrupt contractions of which are usually more painful than those produced naturally by your own body; and perhaps most of all, having confidence in yourself that you do have the power and ability to give birth calmly and naturally. (See also Preparing Your Baby for Birth, p. 114.)

# Preparing Your Baby for Birth

You may prepare yourself for labour and the birth of your baby several weeks
or even months beforehand, practising different birthing positions,
exercises, relaxation regimes and even self-hypnosis.

Mothers often visit the place where they will give birth and check it out thoroughly, if the delivery is not to be at home. But what about the unborn baby?

Most will go from a warm, dim, comfortably padded, close environment into a brightly lit, apparently limitless place. To a just-born baby,

it is also very cold because at birth they emerge—soaking wet—into an air temperature that's so much colder than the womb which has been their home until now. For the first time in their lives, they experience firm, direct and uncomfortable touch (wiping, poking prodding, and needling); they will be suddenly

lifted up, carried about and weighed and measured. They have never before seen or felt anything like this, and nothing in the womb has in any way prepared them for such experiences. For most babies, modern Western-style birth must be a shock (see Being Born—and Welcoming Your Baby, p. 132). However, much

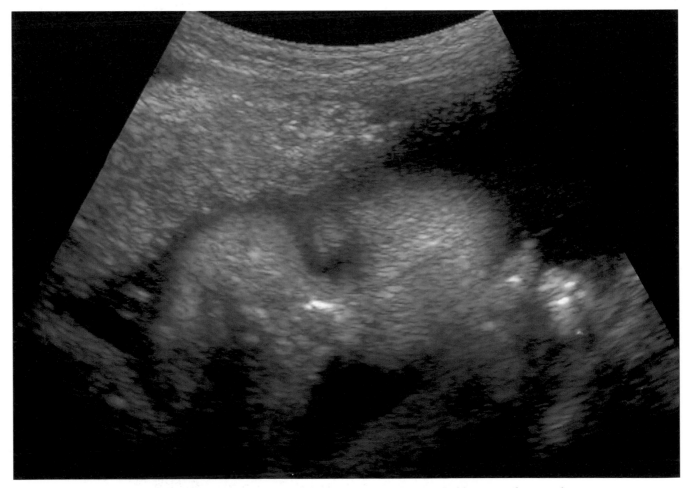

*ABOVE: This full-term foetus's facial features are clearly distinguishable on an ultrasound scan.
Even the baby's chubby cheeks can be seen in the middle of the scan.*

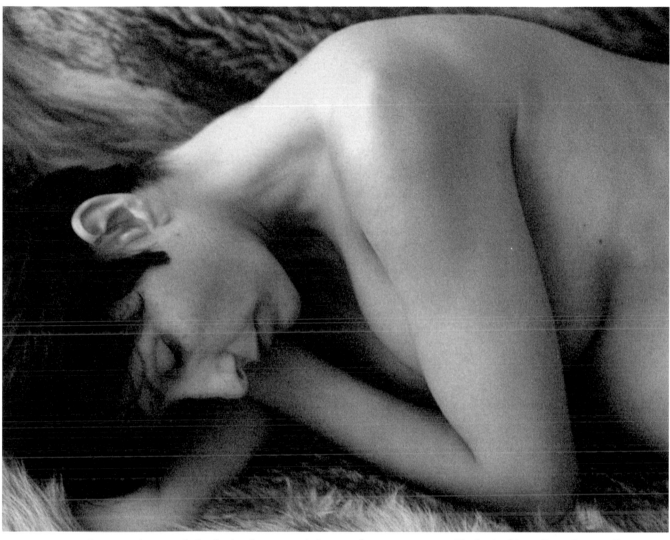

*ABOVE: In preparing your baby for birth it is vital that you first prepare yourself—both physically and mentally.*

as we might want to, we can't reach our babies inside the womb to teach them something about the sensations and experiences that will avalanche over them as soon as they are born.

Or can we? Apparently there are several things a mother-to-be can do to help gently prepare her child for the environment he or she will meet outside the cushioning shelter of the womb. According to Dr. Chairat Panthuraamphorn, the Head of the Prenatal Enrichment Unit at Bangkok's Hua Chiew General Hospital: "The

day of birth comes like an earthquake." His unit has developed an in-womb preparation programme to soften the experience, which expectant mothers can carry out with their unborn babies at home. It includes gently squeezing your own abdomen during the last two months of pregnancy, which may help familiarize your baby with the womb contractions of labour. Involuntary Braxton Hicks practice contractions do a similar job.

Another step is periodically to shine a strong light (perhaps from a

torch) close to your lower abdomen, around where your baby's eyes are. This is thought to help prepare babies for daylight and for the bright lights trained on them in the standard birthing room, and also to stimulate their vision.

Placing a bottle of cold water briefly on your abdomen over the baby's back area is also recommended. This helps the foetus prepare for the coldness that will be felt immediately after birth.

Rhythmic patting and stroking over your abdomen teaches your baby to experience the "birth pat"

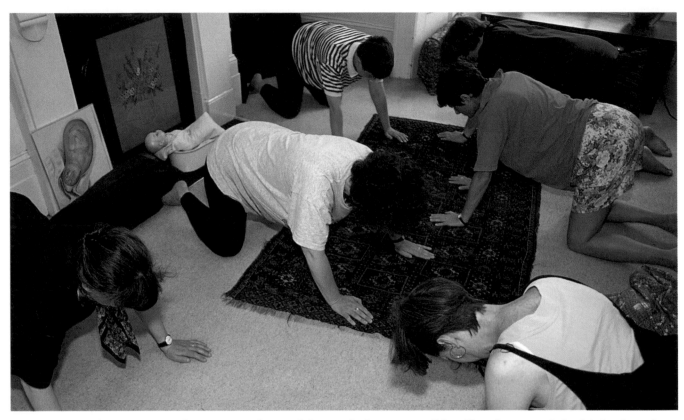

*ABOVE: Gentle exercise is good preparation for your labour, which in turn will be of benefit to your baby. Joining in a class with other pregnant women is a good idea as it gives a feeling of solidarity.*

without alarm (birth pats are those traditional pats or small slaps on a newborn's buttocks intended to encourage its breathing).

Rocking, perhaps in a rocking chair, according to the Bangkok team, prepares the baby for "movements through space... and the rapid motions which occur at birth". They add that the motion also "improves motor tone and balance".

Another step is practising the "training pat". Pat your abdomen each time you feel your baby move inside you. The baby will eventually learn to move in response to your patting. Dr. Panthuraamphorn also suggests that this helps the child learn to respond to outside stimuli and improves the development of muscle tone.

## HELPING YOUR BABY PREPARE FOR THE OUTSIDE WORLD

A mother can help her baby prepare for the shock of coming into the outside world in several ways. Remember that it is a colder, brighter place than your baby's been used to.

*Spraying your abdomen lightly with cold water will help your baby adjust to temperature differences outside the womb.*

*A torch held against your tummy will be registered by your baby and help make the brightness of the delivery room more comfortable.*

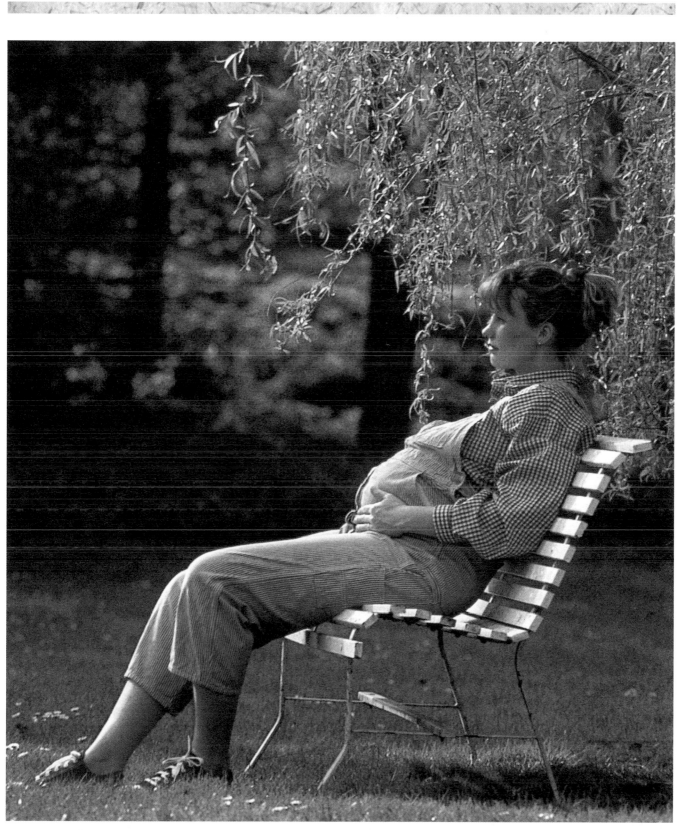

ABOVE: *If you can, in any quieter moments, do some gentle visualization—literally "seeing in your mind's eye" the birth progressing easily and naturally—it can help prepare the way for a smoother, more relaxed labour.*

# Overdue Babies

A normal pregnancy lasts anywhere between 37 and 41 weeks, the classic timespan being 40 weeks.

About one in ten mothers has a pregnancy lasting 40-plus weeks. Childbirth professionals have concerns about pregnancies that are longer than is usual because these are associated with a greater likelihood of problems for the baby, so some obstetricians prefer to avoid the situation by artificially inducing labour. Unfortunately, the latter tends to mean a more medically managed, sometimes more restrictive birth.

*LEFT: Waiting for an overdue baby to be born can be a test of patience for all members of the family.*

## OVERDUE OR NOT

Often, however, a baby is not really overdue at all: it is just that no one knows precisely when pregnancy began. The usual methods rely on the mother having a "standard" 28-day menstrual cycle with ovulation occurring on day 14, and on the mother knowing the date of her last menstrual period or the date she conceived. These calculation techniques are not very accurate, however, because only 8 per cent of women have the classic cycle length. The time of ovulation also varies, and can shift from month to month as well; research studies suggest that on average a third of pregnant women cannot be sure when their last period began.

It is interesting, according to Professor Linda Cardozo, of King's College Hospital, London, that babies are even more likely to be born healthy, and to survive, if they arrive between 41 and 42 weeks, than they are if they are born between 39 and 40 weeks. If they arrive at or after 43 weeks, however, they have twice the risk of death within the first month as the 39- to 40-weekers. It is therefore fine for a pregnancy to continue at its own pace for up to two weeks past an accurately dated due day.

## INDUCING LABOUR

Some obstetricians, however, may suggest inducing your labour if you go seven to ten days past your estimated delivery date, in case your baby is more overdue than everyone

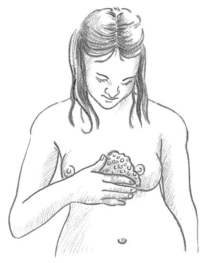

*ABOVE: An endoscope was used to capture this image of a baby, five minutes before birth; the hair on the child's head is clearly visible.*

thinks. Potential problems for overdue babies include: an increased risk of inhaling fragments of their earliest bowel waste (called meconium), which can cause breathing problems after birth; a rapidly decreasing amount of amniotic fluid, which can encourage umbilical cord compression and oxygen shortage either in the womb or during labour; sleep disturbances, illnesses and feeding difficulties after the birth; and a general shortage of oxygen to the foetus, because the supplies to late babies tend to be lower—low enough for the natural, temporary "shut-off" effect of uterine contractions to sometimes cause foetal distress (the medical term used to describe insufficient oxygen getting through).

*ABOVE: Gently sponging your nipples or dripping water on to them is one way a mother-to-be can help the onset of labour. It is thought to release the oxytocin hormone, which brings on womb contractions.*

## LATE BABIES

If your pregnancy extends past the 40-week stage it is reassuring to know that it is certainly not unusual.

• Pregnancies tend to be up to four days longer if they deliver in summer rather than in winter.

• Post-mature babies may have longer hair on their heads than babies born earlier, long fingernails and dry and dull skin; they may be longer, thinner and more alert, and may not have any vernix (a creamy substance often covering the foetus) or lanugo (the fine soft body hair) on their skin.

### YOU CAN ENCOURAGE YOUR OWN LABOUR TO BEGIN BY

• Making love (the semen contains prostaglandins, which encourage womb contractions).

• Stimulating your own nipples for 20 minutes at a time, either by gentle touch or dripping on water from a facecloth. This triggers the release of oxytocin, a hormone which also encourages womb contractions.

• Doing anything that disturbs the intestines a little—eat a hot, spicy meal or take a long walk.

• Having a professional acupuncture or acupressure treatment.

The longest recorded pregnancy was in 1883. It supposedly lasted 476 days, resulting in a 5.8 kg (13-pound) boy. However, the truth of this claim is "very doubtful" according to medical historians.

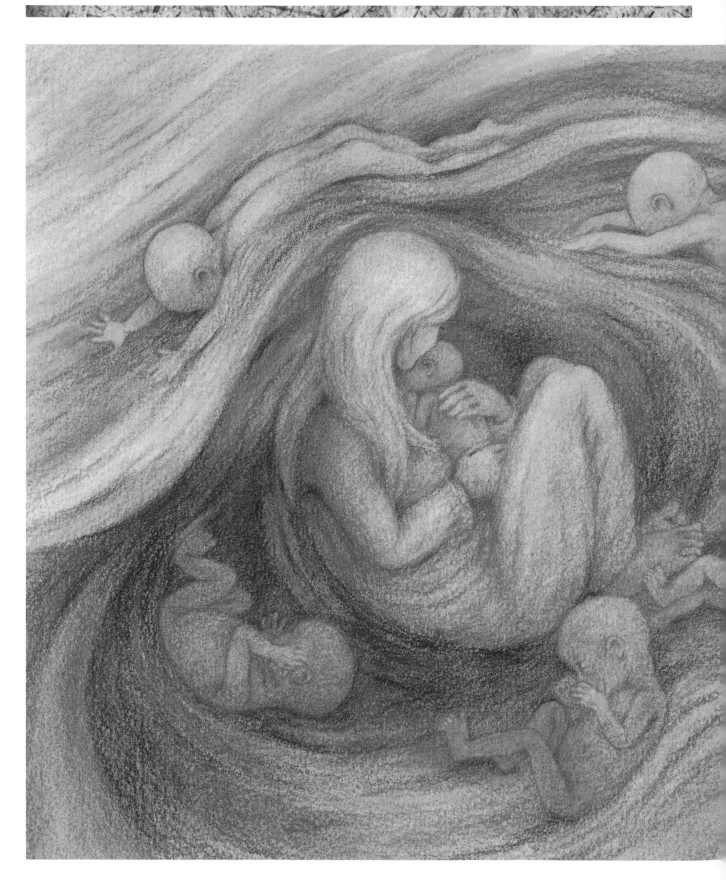

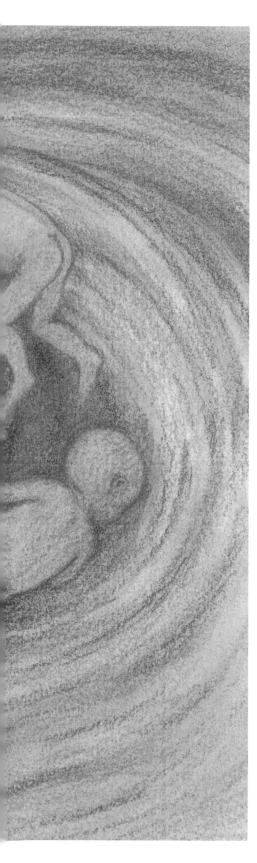

# Memories of Being in the Womb—and Being Born

## Scientists and psychologists have been arguing about whether or not people can really remember their own births—and so what if they do?—for the past 100 years.

The grandfathers of modern psychology came across birth-related flashbacks, dreams and images as early as 1929 (Otto Rank) and in 1933 (Sigmund Freud). New York psychologist Nandor Fodor was conducting birth related dreamwork with his patients in the late 1940s, and Arthur Janov (the founder of primal therapy) in the early 1960s. Yet, birth memories were still thought to be questionable. Are they genuine memories of real importance? If so, why are they important? Sceptics suggest these are just creative fantasies based on fragments of information given to the person years later, examples of "false memory", originating from leading questions made by a therapist, or the result of leading questions and suggestions made to subjects under hypnosis.

### CHANGING ATTITUDES

Until the 1960s, no one except a small contingent of progressive therapists cared much either way. In the late 1990s, however, birth memories are becoming an important issue, because there are a growing number of people from the age of two years and up who seem to be experiencing them. Once only ever heard of as curious one-off reports in fringe magazines, there are now case studies, and published, unbiased research trials (see pp. 154-55) involving many subjects of all ages. One little girl mentions "the yukky white mud on me when I came out of my mother's tummy". My own son asked: "Why was my dressing gown cord around me when I came out?" although I have never told him he was born with the umbilical cord around his neck.

Once thought of as an interesting but esoteric side issue, birth memories are now being seen as vital buried clues as to why we are the way we are. The past 30 years' research into these repressed and often deeply buried memories suggests that even though most people cannot remember their births without help, they certainly act them out throughout childhood and adulthood. A growing number of psychologists and therapists, along with some enlightened obstetricians, are becoming convinced that the way you were born and the first few minutes of life outside the womb have a profound effect upon your personality, and that negative memories can be recovered—and altered—using psychological therapies.

### HELPING PEOPLE REMEMBER

There are many different techniques, including special breathing methods, light or deep hypnosis, guided meditation and fantasy, dreamwork, Gestalt (a German school of psychology which stresses the unity of self-awareness, behaviour, and experience), primal therapy, free association, isolation in flotation tanks and rebirthing therapy sessions. Sometimes the memory surfaces with no help at all as a sudden flashback, a recurring dream, or a puzzling image.

## WHAT THEY REMEMBER

"Today, two-year-old children are blurting out their birth memories invited or uninvited; they present verifiable facts and ask disturbing questions," writes psychologist Dr. David B. Chamberlain, President of the Association for Pre- and Perinatal Psychology and Health.

Psychotherapist Dr. William Emerson, whose speciality is infant birth refacilitation, cites many cases of such birth memories, such as a little girl named Rowan who would regularly push herself into the corner of her cot and lodge her head against the bars. Her parents said her second stage of labour had been very difficult, with Rowan stuck in the birth canal, uncomfortably wedged for $4^1/2$ hours.

A study by Dr. Chamberlain compared reports of ten births obtained under light hypnosis. In each case, he checked the mother's memories against the child's—the latter were between 9 and 23 years old, and had never heard any details about their birth. Their reports were remarkably coherent, with the same story told from two different perspectives. One example is the child whose mother had described herself as drunk and disorientated by anaesthetic drugs, who said: "My mother is not all there. She doesn't seem awake or have her eyes open." Babies

remember what you first say around them, too. Another child remembered just after she was born her mother spoke her name and said "I love you"; her mother's version was she said "I love you", and called her "Michelle". Yet another mother recalled she said, "Oh God! She has deformed toes!" while the child's version was: "She asks the nurse why my toes are so funny..." It also appears babies notice more than their new environment, or even the comments made about them and how they are welcomed. Many interviewees reported that as soon as they were born they felt they were intelligent and fully aware, but had no means of expressing this and found it very frustrating.

## INTELLIGENT PERSONALITIES

Deborah explains what it felt like to come out of the womb and not be able to make herself understood or taken seriously: "I felt I knew a lot, I really did... I never thought of being a person... I thought I was an intelligent mind. They seemed to ignore me, they were doing things to the outside of me, but they acted like that's all there was... I just really felt I was more intelligent than they were." Jeff talks about the peace and delight his mother gave him when he was brought up from the communal baby nursery to her: he knew right away she was someone special: "Somehow I knew I was safe with her, that I had nothing to worry about with this person. When she held me or spoke to me there was just something different. I could tell she cared for me in a way the others did not. She was totally concerned..." (From *The Significance of Birth Memories*, by Dr. David B. Chamberlain.)

## ACTING IT OUT

Prenatal psychologists say we all have buried birth memories, it's just a matter of finding them. Some research suggests adults can also, under regressive hypnosis, show the unique types of behaviour only seen in term foetuses or newborn babies, and which, under usual circumstances, even adult actors cannot replicate. One particular experiment in 1982, by the Russian psychologist Vladimir Raikov, showed that under deep hypnosis, adults spontaneously showed the startle and moro reflexes (which babies lose within weeks of birth), as well as the uncoordinated eye movements that newborns make, rooting and sucking behaviour (see Your Amazing Newborn Baby, p. 142).

The San Franciscan obstetrician Dr. David Cheek also carried out hypnotic work on several adults whom he had delivered when he was a young obstetrician 20 years before, in Chico, California. They were able to demonstrate the exact sequence of turns of their own head and shoulders as they passed down through the birth canal, details they could not possibly have known. The relevant records had all been stored in Dr. Cheek's personal files for the previous two decades. He went on to work with about 500 more adults in a similar way, finding that they could recall their sequence of birth positions and movements—whether they were born in the vertex (head down) position, breech or by Caesarean. Their "muscle memories"—neurological recall of particular types and patterns of movement sequences laid down in the relevant muscle groups—were all accurately reproduced.

## WHAT BABIES REMEMBER OF BIRTH

Dr. Chamberlain finds these memories vary greatly. For one little boy whose mother had had a difficult labour, the experience left him "exhausted, aching and stiff". Yet other children describe being born as "like going down a slide backwards", "like a tidal wave", and "like being in a ship on a rocky sea". One girl, Theresa, remembers: "it's dark... I'm getting a rush of energy... I feel like I'm going to explode! I feel like everything is rushing to my head!" Some aspects of birth can be very rewarding and exciting for newborns, as it involves marvellous first-time discoveries: "Looking at things with my eyes is so much more fun... the more I do it, the more fun it is..." and "My hands and legs move so easily..." According to Laura, remembering looking at all the people in the delivery room: "I feel special, I'm the reason everybody's here... I'm the reason they're smiling. I feel like a present!"

If loving and welcoming comments babies hear at birth stay with them, it also appears, however, that careless words can hurt, and hurt badly. Here is a short list of some remarks made by doctors, nurses and parents at birth, which did, in fact, result in long-term damage for the child, surfacing in therapy with Dr. Chamberlain: "They could lose me—that's what they said... I don't want to go. I haven't been here very long. I'm little." "What's wrong with her head?" "Wow—this looks like a sickly one!" "Another girl—she's skinny." "She's not important, take care of the mother." "Look at her! We're lucky she was born at all with all those things wrong."

## MEMORIES FROM THE WOMB

Under hypnosis, children and adults can also recall events that happened when they were still in the womb. Some of these memories are visual. Others are emotional. These memories of the womb can also be acted out later, and can be especially noticeable in the way twins behave towards each other first inside, then outside, the womb (see Twins and You, p. 104).

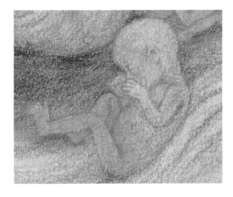

Dr. Chamberlain also tells the story of one of his patients, a mother with a small baby who found she was "half-waking up at night in great distress, asking: 'Where's the baby? Where's the baby?' She was never reassured when her husband would say to her quite truthfully 'But our baby's right here in the crib.' Unconvinced, she would sleepwalk through all the rooms, even wander up and down the street at night searching for this baby. When she came to see me she was on the verge of being sent to a psychiatric hospital. Yet, in her first hypnosis session she was able to identify a twin who had died while they were both in her mother's womb, and how deeply this still upset her. That was the baby she was searching for. To me, this sort of case history strongly suggests pre-

nates have strong, clear impressions and memories."

After working with more than 1,000 subjects in three- to six-day residential courses around the world, British psychiatrist and rebirthing expert Frank Lake was also convinced that the first three months in the womb are the origin of conditions as diverse as asthma, migraine and food allergy, as well as certain personality disorders.

Explanations of how a memory is planted when someone is a foetus only a few inches long and with a rudimentary brain are varied, but they include the idea of cellular memory (prebirth memory). This coincides with Karl Pribam's idea that the brain records images holographically, allowing pictures of the whole to be distributed and stored in all its different parts, and the newer "wet brain" thesis, in which the brain is a gland operating with hormones and fluids.

## WHY BIRTH MEMORIES MATTER

Being born is a major event which happens to every single one of us. If birth memories actually exist, influence the way we live and affect our personalities for better or worse, they are an important and powerful part of our psychological make-up.

But perhaps the best news of all is that birth memories are something all future parents can influence positively, for their own children. We do not have to repeat the mistakes previous generations have made. We can, by making the transition of newborns into our world as gentle, loving and respectful as possible, help ensure that their first—and lasting—impressions are good ones.

# Labour—What to Expect

Labour is the natural process by which women bring their babies into the world. No two labours are alike.

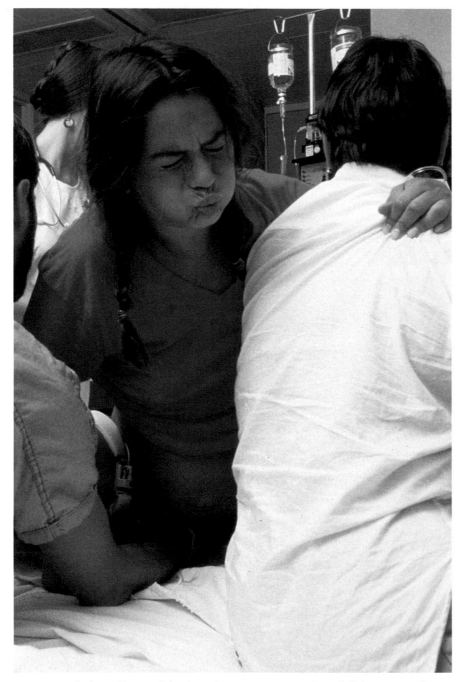

*ABOVE: Labour "proper" begins when your contractions fall into a regular pattern, then become closer together. The sensations begin in the small of your back and radiate right around to the front, just above your pubic bone.*

Labour usually follows a general pattern of three—many would say four—distinct stages. First-time births tend to take longer, between seven and nine hours, but subsequent births are faster, between four and five hours. Again, there is a wide range of normality, as some babies arrive within an hour, and yet other mothers can be in labour for 24 hours or even more.

### FIRST STAGE

Your womb muscles contract, or clench, powerfully, gradually making the womb smaller, and pulling up and dilating the cervix (the neck of the womb). The cervix, which has remained faithfully closed throughout pregnancy and kept your baby safely in the womb, needs to dilate until there is a gap just less than 10 cm (4 inches) wide; this is also the diameter of the baby's head circumference at its narrowest angle of presentation. By the end of the first stage your body will have created a birth canal—the temporary, single passage of open womb, open cervix, and vagina—down which your baby can pass to be born.

### WHILE YOU'RE IN LABOUR

Stay as calm and as focused as you can: relaxation techniques, slow breathing, warm water and the support of a partner and birth attendant you trust all help. Hold on to your confidence in your own body's instinctive ability to give birth—generally bodies do know how, and manage it extraordinarily well, so attempt to go with what you think yours is telling you.

Try to experience as much of your labour as possible in positions which help keep you upright. This gives you the advantage of gravity working with you, rather than against you, to help you push your baby out more easily. Do whatever feels most comfortable for you and keep changing your position to suit how you are feeling. Options women say they find especially useful include standing and leaning against your partner or birth attendant while he or she massages your lower back; sitting and leaning over a chair back, bean bag or pile of pillows; squatting between your partner's or birth attendant's knees while he or she supports you under your arms and against your back; kneeling on all fours for a while; walking about slowly whenever possible; semi-reclining; or relaxing in a birthing pool, ordinary warm bath or shower.

## WHAT DOES CHILDBIRTH FEEL LIKE?

Labour pains are called contractions. They will probably begin by feeling merely uncomfortable—women often say they feel just like strong period pains—becoming steadily stronger and more uncomfortable as labour progresses. Labour pain does not come directly from your womb, but is due to ischaemia, a lack of blood in the uterine muscles produced by the womb working hard. This hurts for the same reason that a heart attack or angina hurts: lack of oxygen to the muscles, and a build-up of cellular waste products which irritate nerve tissue.

*RIGHT: Gentle yoga exercises can be a marvellous way to relax as you approach labour.*

## POSITIONS FOR AN EASIER LABOUR

Between contractions it helps enormously if you can consciously and deliberately relax. Try using deep, slow breathing—in for a count of 8, hold it for 8, then slowly breathe out for 8. This is: easy, even if you have not practised it before; less complicated than the breathing techniques taught in antenatal classes; and remarkably rapid in producing a soothing, calming effect. It's also important to adopt a position that makes you feel as comfortable as possible. Here are some options that women have found especially helpful.

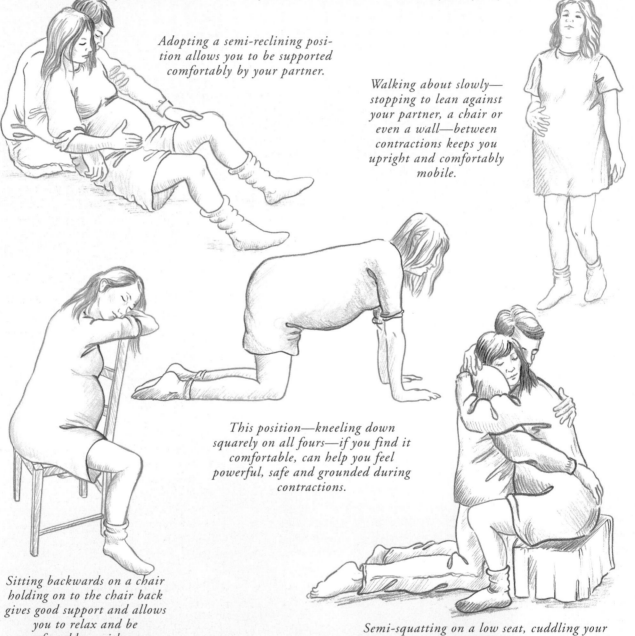

*Adopting a semi-reclining position allows you to be supported comfortably by your partner.*

*Walking about slowly—stopping to lean against your partner, a chair or even a wall—between contractions keeps you upright and comfortably mobile.*

*This position—kneeling down squarely on all fours—if you find it comfortable, can help you feel powerful, safe and grounded during contractions.*

*Sitting backwards on a chair holding on to the chair back gives good support and allows you to relax and be comfortable—without a partner needing to be there too.*

*Semi-squatting on a low seat, cuddling your partner, gives you physical support and emotional encouragement, and helps keep you in the best position for labour—upright.*

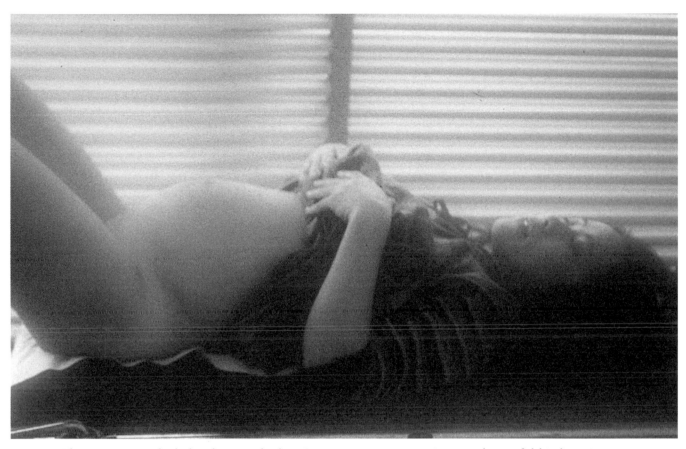

*ABOVE: If you can, turn the lights down and relax. By creating your own private and peaceful birth environment, even in a hospital room, you can turn your thoughts inward to concentrate on your birth and exclude outside distractions.*

However, labour is different from ordinary types of pain because it behaves differently, and it is therefore easier to tolerate. Labour pain begins slowly and gently, builds up to a peak, then recedes. Then there is a rest from 20 or 30 minutes, if you are in very early labour, to a minute or two towards the end, before another contraction begins. This lets you get your breath and balance back. It is also unique in that it is happening for a very positive reason—giving birth to your baby. The pain can almost always be coped with or relieved to some extent and sometimes totally obliterated, using gentler, natural methods of pain relief, or powerful analgesic drugs.

### TRANSITION

Many obstetricians say this is not a stage as such, but others explain it as the time when the womb changes the way it is contracting—from spasms which are making the womb progressively smaller and dilating the cervix, to the powerful expulsive type of contractions which push your baby out. Some women do not notice any change, but others report feeling irritable, impatient and angry with their partners or birth attendants; muddled and confused; suddenly unable to cope, at the end of their patience; sick, shaky or cold; or lost because their formerly regular contractions suddenly seem to have no proper pattern to them.

### SECOND STAGE

This is sometimes called the "pushing stage", as it is exactly what you are doing. This stage takes anything from 30 minutes to 2 or 3 hours, but may happen in as little as 5 minutes. Many women report a surge of excitement and an extra burst of energy now; others remember an irresistible urge to "bear down" (push).

There are, in fact, three phases here. During the first, your baby emerges from the bony cradle of your pelvis, pushed around at an angle into your vagina, with its head and shoulders rotating gracefully. During the second phase, your womb continues contracting strongly, each one helping to move the baby a small part of

## THE STAGES OF LABOUR

Labour falls into four (some say three) different stages. The duration of
each stage and hence the timing of the overall labour varies greatly—for
some women it can take 24 hours or more.

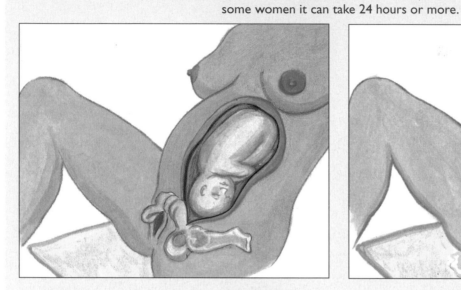

*Stage 1, early: the muscle contractions of your womb
begin to make the space smaller, pulling up and opening
out the cervix (neck of the womb) to form the baby's
doorway into the vagina.*

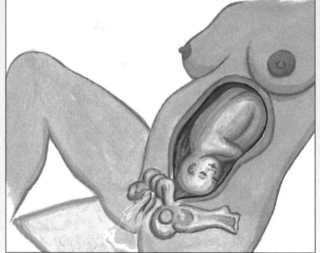

*Stage 2 (phase 1): this is called the pushing stage because
that is just what you are now doing to ease your baby
down the birth canal. This usually takes 30 to 60
minutes, but it can last as long as a couple of hours.*

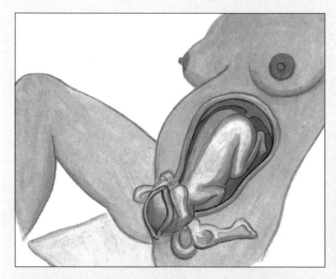

*Stage 2 (phase 2): the cervix has been effaced to create the
birth canal—a single passageway of womb, open cervix
and vagina, down which your baby can now pass to be
born. This can last for 6 to 24 hours, but the average for
first babies is 7 to 9 hours, and 4 to 5 hours for
subsequent births.*

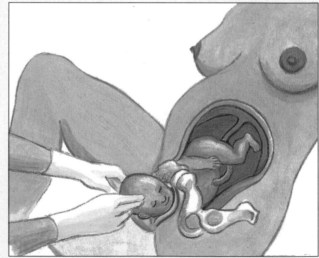

*Stage 3 (phase 3): the birth itself. Your baby is pushed
out of the birth canal and into the outside world.
(Not shown: the delivery of the placenta, which may take
only a few minutes if you have had an injection to speed
up the process, or up to half an hour or more if it is
allowed to happen naturally.)*

## THE SECRET OF BIRTH

Many women wonder how something the size of a baby can possibly pass down somewhere as narrow as their vagina.

It is possible, however, because the vagina expands remarkably: inside, it is made up of many folds of elastic tissue, which become even more elastic due to the relaxing effect of extra progesterone during the 40 weeks of pregnancy. The other secret is that a vagina stretches slowly, gently and steadily. It will return within virtually a matter of weeks to its pre-pregnancy dimensions.

In about half of all births, the perineum (the muscular area between the vagina and the anal opening) tears slightly to allow the baby's head past, or the midwife or obstetrician may make a small sterile scissor cut, called an episiotomy, for the same purpose. You will probably feel neither because of the intense stretching in the area, and any cuts will be stitched, if necessary, immediately after the birth.

the way along the birth canal. During the third phase, your baby is pushed out of the birth canal's exit and into the world.

As your baby emerges from the birth canal, the narrowest part of his or her head is usually leading the way, and where the head has passed, the rest of the body follows easily. When the face first comes into contact with the air, the change in temperature usually stimulates the baby to take a first breath and fill the lungs—so even before he or she is fully "out" you may hear the first protesting or surprised cry. Some

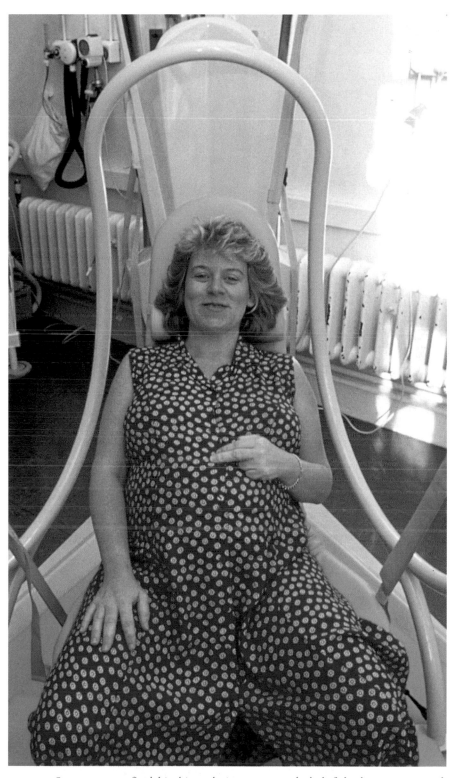

*ABOVE: Some women find birthing chairs enormously helpful; there are several designs, from a V-shaped floor cushion in a rigid frame to more complicated versions like this one, but they all help keep you in the best position for most births—a supported, comfortable, upright, semi-squatting position.*

A survey was conducted of 100 new mothers at St. George's Hospital, in London, to find out what labour felt like. Their descriptions include:

"I just thought I had indigestion."

"An intermittent heavy period pain-like ache in my lower back."

"Not painful, but I felt like my stomach was heaving."

"Stabbing pains across my lower abdomen."

"Like being very constipated."

"A dull ache in my lower back."

Comments also varied from "no one ever told me it could be that bad" and "unbelievably painful" to "I don't see what all the fuss was about", "totally exhilarating and really exciting", "almost orgasmic at the end", and "really hard physical work, but not painful as such".

babies, however, such as many of those born by the Leboyer method (which uses massage, relaxation and the minimum of intervention during labour, and welcomes the baby with dimmed lights, quiet voices, a warm-water bath and immediate

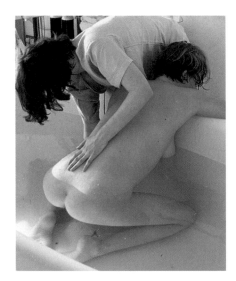

*ABOVE: A combination of gentle massage and the support of water can help ease labour pains.*

breast-feeding) have been born, according to Frederick Leboyer himself, smiling serenely.

### THIRD STAGE

By now you will probably be cuddling your new baby and it may be suckling from your breast, so you may not be especially aware of anything else happening. But there is one final stage—delivery of the placenta. As your womb contracts and shrinks, the placenta attached to it crumples and peels off. Initially this exposes the blood vessels that have been supplying your baby in the womb, but they close down rapidly as the womb continues to become smaller. The placenta is painlessly shed out through your vagina by the next few contractions. If you have been given an injection of synthetic oxytocin to speed up the process, it only takes a few minutes, otherwise it can take up to half an hour or so.

ABOVE: *Mothers often describe the first contact with their newborn to be like falling in love for the first time.*

BELOW: *Holding her baby in her arms for the first time is a precious moment for any new mother.*

## PAIN RELIEF IN LABOUR—WHAT WORKS BEST?

The following are some of the most popular and widely available methods of pain relief in labour. Their effectiveness scores, based on the percentage of mothers describing it as "good" or "very good" in the UK's National Birthday Trust survey of 1993, are given.

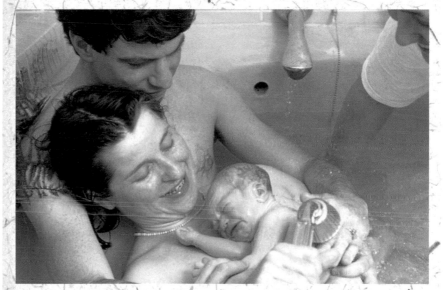

ABOVE: *Water can have a remarkably soothing effect for women in labour, their partners and their babies too. It can provide a good measure of pain relief, precious intimacy and privacy—rare in modern hospital childbirths.*

### METHODS OF PAIN RELIEF

- Nitrous oxide and oxygen—more commonly simply called gas and air (85 per cent)

- Pethidine/Demerol (71 percent)

- Epidural (94 per cent)

- Water (no figures; however, according to Janet Balaskas, founder of *the Active Birth Movement*, in the UK: "Pain does remain challenging, but is easier to cope with.")

- Massage (90 per cent)

- Relaxation and breathing techniques (89 per cent)

- TENS (transcutaneous electrical nerve stimulation) units, which give very mild electrical stimulation to mask pain (up to 75 per cent)

- Self-hypnosis and autogenic training—a system of deep physical and mental relaxation, which can put you in a state of light self-hypnosis (no firm figures are available, but labours take approximately one-third less time, and require less usual pain relief)

- Acupuncture (two-thirds of women found this "useful")

- Aromatherapy (62 per cent)

# Being Born—and Welcoming Your Baby

"You can't say a newborn doesn't speak. It's we who do not listen," according to Dr. Frederick Leboyer, obstetrician. However, no one can ask a baby at the time how it was for him or her—not in words, anyway.

Comments from women just after they have given birth include: "exciting", "triumphant", "very painful", "exhilarating", "exhausting", "terrifying", "hours of calm progression building up to 15 minutes when all hell was let loose", "really hard work—they don't call it labour for nothing", "a titanic physical struggle", and "well, I don't understand what all the fuss is about".

According to the psychologist Arthur Janov, founder-director of the world-famous Primal Therapy Institute, in California, and formerly with the psychiatric department of the Los Angeles Children's Hospital and the State of California Narcotics Outpatient Program, babies' very earliest and most intense experiences are laid down deep in their memory banks, and, if necessary, can be recovered later in psychotherapy, often using regressive hypnosis. This is a gentle technique which allows the child or adult to be guided, as if going backwards in time through memories of infancy, babyhood, birth and even back as far as the time spent in the womb. "Birth… is the first prolonged emotional and physical shock the child undergoes," writes top Toronto pre-

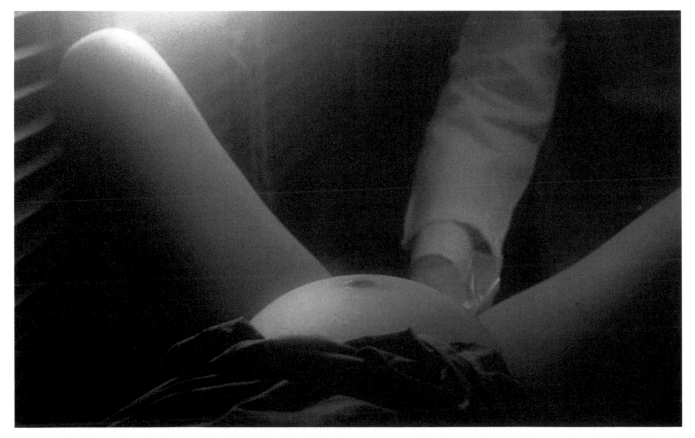

*ABOVE: A helping hand supports the baby's head as it begins to emerge. Birth attendants will sometimes lay their hand against the mother's perineum to provide gentle but firm counterpressure to the area so it does not tear.*

and perinatal psychologist Dr. Thomas Verny, "and he (the baby) never quite forgets it".

## SO WHY DO WE FORGET?

Mothers often find their memories of giving birth fade over time (sometimes within only a few months). The babies tend not to have any recall of the experience unless carefully prompted by hypnosis or rebirthing therapy in later childhood or adulthood. But why do we forget an experience as intense and as important as this so easily? According to Dr. Verny, it is probably because of a hormone called oxytocin, which is released in large quantities during childbirth by the mother to encourage her womb to contract. In animal experiments, oxytocin has been found to induce amnesia.

But the experiences are there, even if they are buried. There are hundreds of such individual reminiscences and small groups of documented case histories of adults' very individual birth memories. No two are alike, just as no two births are alike, yet there are also recurring themes and some general similarities, initially identified in research carried out by the psychiatrist Dr. Stanislav Grof. He conducted several hundred interviews after the interviewees had been given LSD as a means of opening up the subconscious. The full collection was published in a book called *The Realms of the Human Unconscious*, in 1975, in which Grof divides birth experiences into four stages termed the Basic Perinatal Matrices. The memories run the full range—from a blissful, calm euphoria and a feeling of being completely at one with the environment and the

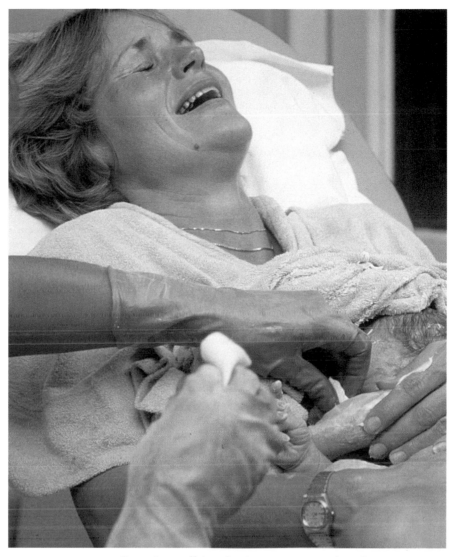

*ABOVE: Sometimes all it takes is one more good push...*

universe (the latter is also a common positive reaction to an LSD trip), to flashbacks of suffocation and fear of death. Listed here are the four stages he identified.

### Prelabour

Bliss, calm, a sense of freedom in which to make oneself comfortable, to kick freely and to push. Dr. Grof thinks that these types of memories tend to correspond with being safely inside the mother's body. They might go way back to the earlier

months of pregnancy, too, because of the feeling of space which the interviewees mentioned, since in the last few weeks conditions become cramped inside the womb.

### First Stage of Labour

Feelings of "I cannot find my way out", of helplessness, of being stuck and of being unable to move—the former freedom has gone and there is nowhere to turn. Dr. Grof described this as the "No Exit" feeling.

## Being Pushed Down the Birth Canal

Interviewees often mentioned a titanic struggle to get out, a sense of a battle between death and being reborn again and at times even a "volcanic ecstasy".

## Birth Itself

Feelings of "enormous decompression", "expansions of space", and "visions of gigantic halls filled with bright radiant light and colour", which perhaps represent having what feels like the limitless space of a brightly lit delivery room around you after having been squashed in the dark of the birth canal for a period of several hours.

Some subjects also recalled being very cold, which may be because babies in the womb inhabit an environment much warmer than the outside world but are born soaking wet and unable to control their own body temperature, so they get very cold rapidly. They often mentioned "a sharp pain in their navel" and being unable to breathe. The latter may be because babies have to learn to breathe as soon as they are born, filling and expelling air from their lungs for the first time. Although they have been practising chest movements in the womb since they were 18 weeks old, the practice never included taking air into their lungs. This rapid changeover may be quite stressful for some, especially if their noses or mouths are temporarily blocked with mucus. Interviewees also mentioned remembering a fear that they were dying, which may go back to feeling unable to breathe.

### WHAT DOES BIRTH FEEL LIKE FOR MOTHERS?

In a 1995 study by midwives at St. George's Hospital, in London (for the book *Pain Relief in Labour*, by Nikki Bradford and Professor Geoffrey Chamberlain), descriptions of first-stage labour contractions included: "Familiar—and so not alarming to me as they felt like increasingly strong period pains which regularly came and went"; "slicing, side-swiping pains low down in my tummy"; "an intermittent sick, low backache"; "I just thought I had indigestion"; "sharp pains that travelled down my inner thighs and across the top of my pubic area"; and "it felt like bad wind, that was all". Severity ranged from "perfectly manageable, except for the last few minutes when I did not know what to do with myself", and "really hard physical work, but I still wouldn't have called it painful as such", to "Excruciating. No one ever told me it was this bad."

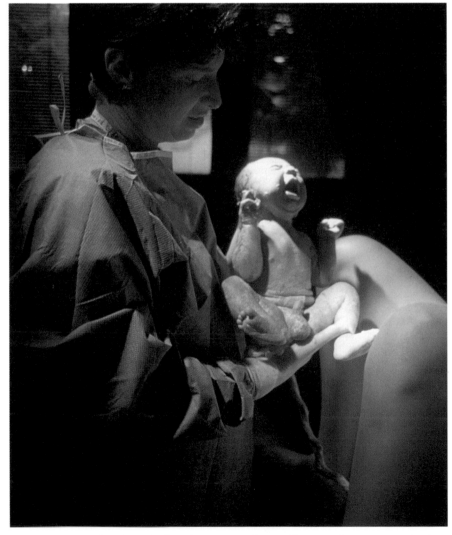

*ABOVE: Giving birth in the familiar surroundings of her own home can make the mother feel more relaxed. In this picture, a newborn baby boy is being held by a doctor just seconds after birth.*

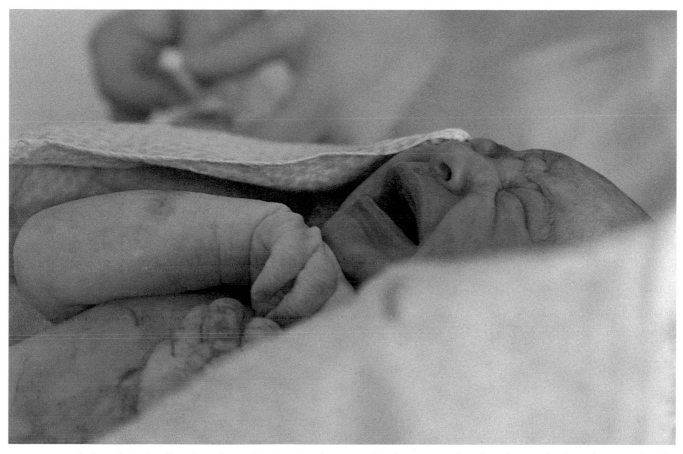

ABOVE: *A baby taking its first breaths and giving its first cry—birth guru Frederick Leboyer also has photographs of babies that have been born calm, even smiling, after gentle, natural births.*

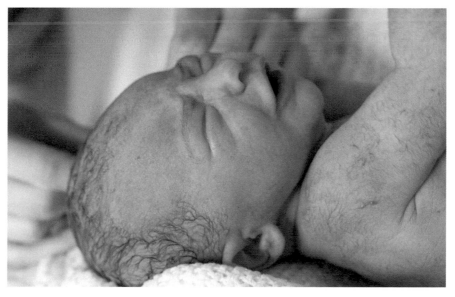

ABOVE: *This baby was born just a couple of minutes before this photograph was taken. Already he has taken his first strong breaths and is beginning to purse his lips and search for his mother's breast.*

135

Of the birth itself: "a burning feeling down there. I think I was too stretched to feel much down there by this time"; "like squeezing toothpaste out of a huge tube"; "like passing a melon out of my bowels"; and "a splitting, tearing sensation". Of the emotions: "excited—I knew this was it"; "reaching down inside myself for extra energy and power I never thought I would find, I was so tired—and finding it"; "one last desperate effort"; "enormous triumph and elation"; and "very fed up. I'd had it. And furious with all these stupid people standing around, shouting at me to push."

### WHAT DOES BIRTH FEEL LIKE FOR BABIES?

Sensations often mentioned under regression therapy or hypnosis include: being squeezed, pushed and squashed; sometimes discomfort and pain in the neck, head or shoulder area, especially if the baby was stuck for a while, or delivered with the help of steel forceps or ventouse suction equipment. (Pulling out a stuck 3.1 kg [7-pound] baby would mean that about 18 kg [40 pounds] of force is exerted on the baby's head and neck.)

Professor Nicholas Fisk, of the Institute of Obstetrics at Queen Charlotte's Hospital, in London, who is researching the possibility that babies may, like many mothers, need pain relief during birth, and if they do, what form it must take and how it could be given, suggests that: "The birth process must feel like being inside a gigantic blood-pressure cuff which covers you from head to toe, squeezing rhythmically on and off. This may be uncomfortable for babies, but it also does fulfil a very important biological function for them as it stimulates the lungs to work and helps complete the maturation process. This is probably why babies who do not experience vaginal birth and who were delivered by Caesarean instead often have difficulty breathing unaided at first."

In addition, many prenatal psychologists also think the physical sensations a baby feels when he or she is born vaginally play an important role in the later development of their sexuality and sensuality. In *The Secret Life of the Unborn Child,* Dr. Verny writes: "Many mothers experience strong sexual feeling during birth, and many of their babies also have moments of intense pleasure as they pass down the birth canal. This is the child's first physical contact—remember they have been submerged in a protective pool of amniotic fluid for the past nine months...

"Now suddenly their entire body is being squeezed, rubbed. Their skin is being directly stimulated for the very first time... (the baby) is also experiencing pain... This combination of pain and pleasure leaves a lasting mark on their sexual inclinations. Generally speaking, the more pleasure a baby experiences during birth, the more likely he or she is to develop normal sexual attitudes later."

### WELCOMING YOUR BABY GENTLY INTO THE WORLD

If being born is a shock to the baby's system, it's also good to know that there is a great deal that both the parents and the birthing staff can do,

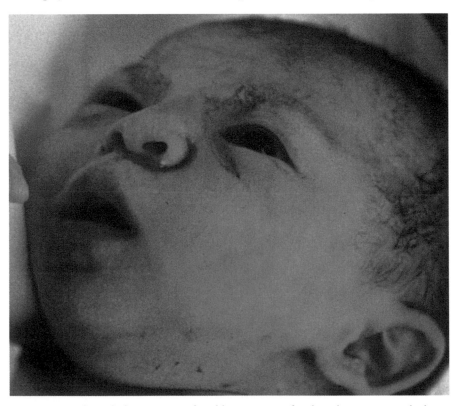

*ABOVE: Newborn babies may not be able to see very far, but they arrive with their vision primed for focusing the exact distance from your breast to your face.*

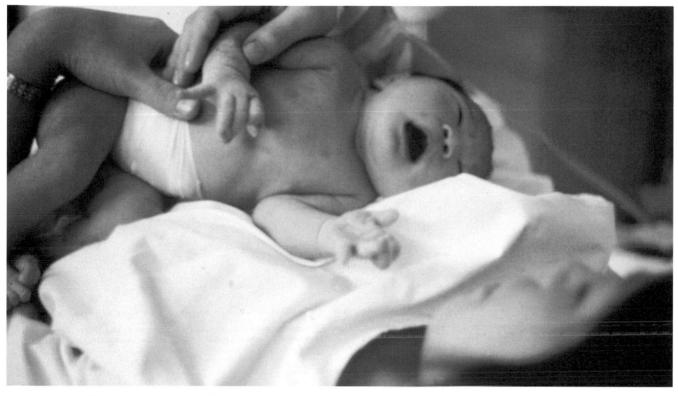

*ABOVE: This newborn baby has been gently washed, weighed and put in a nappy—and is just about to be swathed in a soft blanket and placed in his mother's arms.*

even in the most high-tech of hospital delivery suites, to help make the transition from the womb to the outside world easier.

In Europe, the pioneering work of the French obstetrician Dr. Frederick Leboyer led the way in France. First in France, then in the United Kingdom, Dr. Michel Odent has campaigned for gentler, more respectful birth; both the Active Birth and the water birth movements have done the same in the United Kingdom. In Thailand, top Bangkok obstetrician Dr. Chairat Panthuraamphorn has developed a similar programme, outlined below. Based on simple measures to provide some continuity between the womb environment and the outside world, and owing a good deal to the pioneering work of Leboyer, Dr.

Panthuraamphorn's programme is used at Bangkok's Hua Chiew General Hospital. If it strikes a chord with you, but you feel you might not have the presence of mind to ask while you are giving birth—and who has?—mention the system in your birth plan, so you can discuss it with your obstetrician, nurse or midwife long before the birth. Many of the measures can also be used for a non-emergency Caesarean.

Switch off any air-conditioning before your baby arrives.

Dim bright lights. Low lighting contributes to calm and improves blood pressure and circulation.

Keep sound levels low. Babies are used to sound that is muffled and mediated by the layers of your abdomen and womb.

If possible, cuddle your baby immediately after the birth. Stroke him or her gently and talk softly.

Arrange in advance for a warm bath for your baby soon after birth. This will help recreate the familiar, warm, watery environment of the womb, and gently encourage him or her to adjust to the new surroundings of air.

Ask the staff to wrap your baby loosely for both warmth and free arm and leg movement, then lay him or her on your tummy as soon as possible to be comforted by your familiar heartbeat and breathing rhythms.

Breast-feed right away if you can. This is both calming and bonding because your baby can feel and smell your skin, and suckle, a sensation familar from sucking his or her fingers while in your womb.

# Caesarean Birth

## A Caesarean section is a safe, common operation. In England and Wales, 15 per cent of mothers now have their babies this way; in the United States the rate is 25 per cent.

Physically, a Caesarean is safer for the baby, especially if the child is delicate or premature, but it is still a major medical procedure for the mother.

### WHAT'S INVOLVED?

The operation involves an obstetrician making an incision through the abdominal wall and then through the womb, and lifting the baby out. This part of the process only takes about 10 minutes. These incisions are then stitched separately and very carefully, which takes about 40 minutes.

A C-section, as it is often called, can usually be carried out under an epidural anaesthetic if it has been planned beforehand (an elective Caesarean) or when the procedure is unplanned but there is still enough time to set up the epidural and wait for it to take effect. This way you can be a real part of the event, fully awake to listen to the doctor's and nurse's encouraging commentary on what they are doing, have your partner with you (if you both wish), see your baby being lifted from your womb, and hold, or even breastfeed, him or her virtually right away. Mothers have described the sensa-

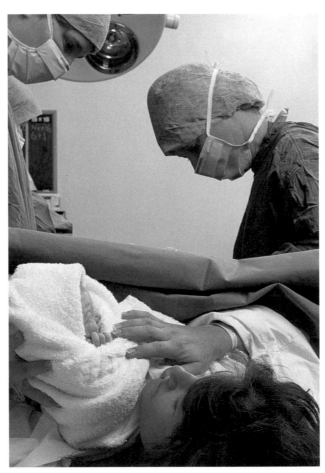

*ABOVE: When you have a Caesarean, the birth itself only takes 10 minutes, though the careful resuturing afterwards takes another 40. If you are having a C-section by epidural, a screen is set up so you can see your baby being lifted out, but not the operation itself.*

tion of the baby being lifted out as "a rummaging feeling, as if someone was doing their washing in there", and "a tugging, pulling sensation, but not at all uncomfortable". If the delivery is an emergency and time is short, a Caesarean will

be done under general anaesthesia. When you wake up, you will probably feel groggy for 24 to 48 hours from the anaesthetic, and so will your baby, but you will probably not remember the operation.

### WHY A CAESAREAN?

One reason for having an emergency Caesarean is that the baby may have become short of oxygen. This is known as foetal distress, and may be due to the physical stress of labour on the baby, a problem with the placenta or the umbilical cord becoming compressed. Signs of distress include a rapid foetal heartbeat.

Another possible reason is that the mother is having irregular or ineffective contractions. Experienced birthing staff should be able to tell the difference between a naturally slow labour, that is, one progressing at its own rate, and one which is barely moving and needs major medical intervention.

You may have an elective Caesarean if you have had any previous babies this way. Other reasons include physical problems relating to the baby. He or she may be lying in an awkward position for birth,

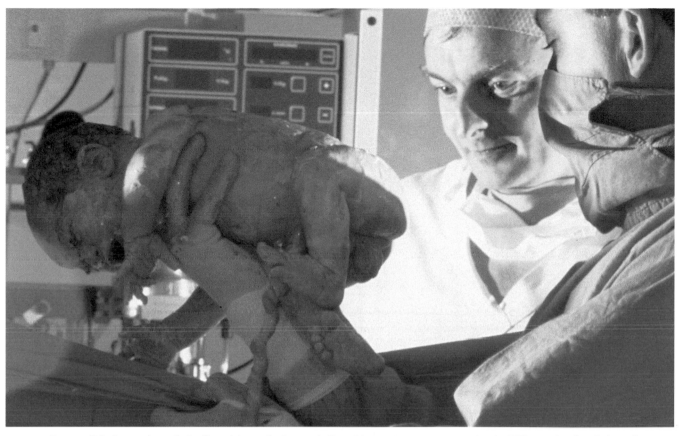

*ABOVE: Doctors lift the newborn baby from his mother's womb. Roughly one in seven women in the UK now has her babies this way.*

such as breech (bottom first), or the head may be too large to pass easily through your pelvis (cephalopelvic disproportion). Certain health problems for the mother often make a Caesarean necessary. These include diabetes (which can mean the baby is very large), very high blood pressure, pre-eclampsia, being HIV-positive or having active genital herpes.

### YOUR CAESAREAN-BORN BABY

Caesarean babies may well feel shock when they arrive so abruptly into a new world, highly conscious of being sharply separated from their mothers, whose bodies they have shared for so long, and very vulnerable to the change of temper-

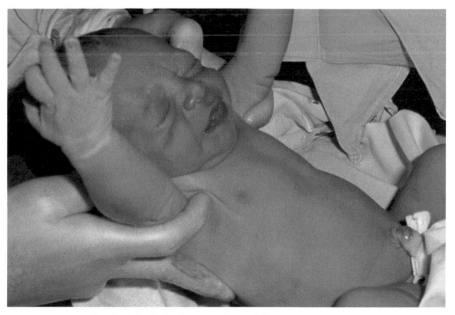

*ABOVE: This healthy baby has just been delivered by Caesarean section, and its umbilical cord clamped. The medical staff will wrap the child gently and warmly before giving her to her mother to hold.*

ature, bright lights or the sensation of being handled. They have never been touched before and have not been neurologically prepared for it by the squeezing of womb contractions. A vaginally born baby also has its breathing mechanisms stimulated by these contractions, but a C-baby does not have the benefit of this, and many have initial breathing problems. This means they may experience the added stress from struggling for breath and having to be medically resuscitated.

Unless there are any good medical reasons preventing it, it helps and reassures a C-baby considerably if you can do what is probably your instinct now anyway—hold and suckle the baby right away and then offer some reassurance by keeping him or her constantly close, perhaps lying on your upper chest (not on your abdomen; it will be sore from the operation) or by your side, touching you.

## WHAT HAPPENS WHEN YOU HAVE AN EPIDURAL?

Some women feel nervous at the thought of having an epidural. It helps to know what's involved before you decide whether or not to have one.

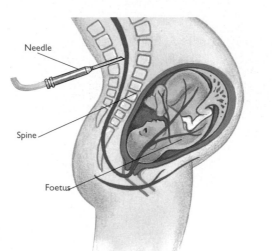

An epidural injection is an effective method of pain relief during labour. A needle is inserted into the woman's back and a local anaesthetic fed through during early labour. This numbs the lower body and helps ease the pain. Some women prefer not to have an epidural, however, as they feel it prevents them from experiencing the birth fully.

Needle

Spine

Foetus

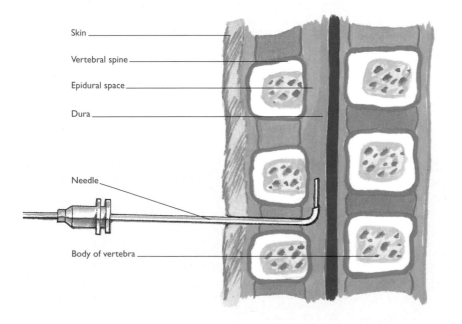

Skin

Vertebral spine

Epidural space

Dura

Needle

Body of vertebra

### EFFECTS OF CAESAREAN DELIVERY

Dr. Arthur Janov, a world-famous psychiatrist, and Director of the Primal Institute in Los Angeles, California, is one of many professionals who believe the events of your birth are indelibly imprinted upon the subconscious, where they are repressed, but relived as feelings, dreams and behaviour in childhood and adulthood: "The earliest pains such as the trauma of birth... are laid down in the very innermost brain structures down into the lower brain stem. They are gated (repressed) by a neurochemical mechanism that keeps those pains from even second-level consciousness."

Regression therapists and psychologists or psychiatrists using rebirthing techniques also say different types of birth can influence behaviour patterns; Dr. Jane English writes that Caesarean and non-Caesarean births "teach you different things. A non-labour Caesarean takes about two minutes—things change totally, suddenly and abruptly. You're here—then suddenly you're there. Something external got you from there to here, you didn't do it for

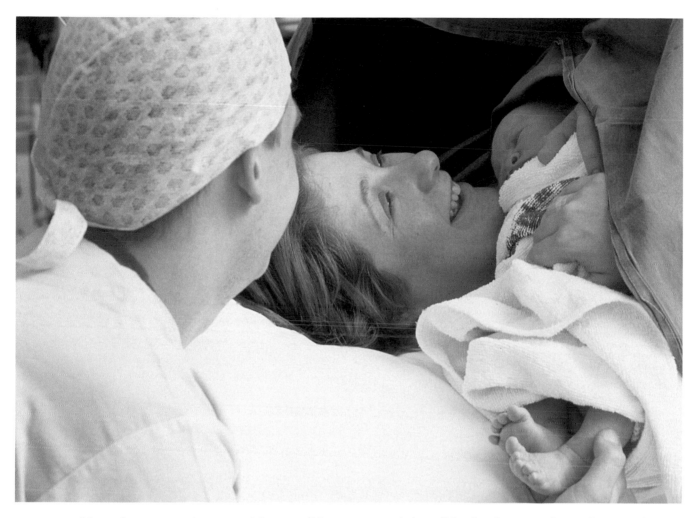

*ABOVE: After a Caesarean section, your abdomen will be sore, so your baby will be placed on your chest or by your side.*

yourself... The lesson is that to get from here to there in future you look outside yourself and find something that will help move you... by comparison, in vaginal birth there is a lesson that there is a slow process... lots of warning, lots of sense that something is changing. The lesson is that you do some work, then there is rest."

She adds: "In vaginal birth you are constricted... Many Caesarean people get 'put in their place' later in life by people who expect them to have this inborn sense of limits which they don't have, as it wasn't part of their birth learning... they

are often told not to be so intrusive, with a lot of negative judgements."

Some of the common general tendencies from Caesarean-born adults may affect the emotional relationships and needs they have. Studies suggest these can include having "rescue fantasies", feeling confused, and according to Dr. Thomas Verny, a psychiatrist in Toronto and founding President of the Association for Pre- and Perinatal Psychology and Health, having "unusually strong desires for touch and sex".

Dr. English also believes that C-people are prone to neck tension

because of their "being pulled rather than pushed at birth", have "relationship patterns that are colourful, abrupt and intense", and have "little sense of process", that is, for them either a relationship exists and does not need to be nourished, or it does not exist, and therefore is impossible. Her work has also led her to believe that they also have a tendency to "trust that help will always be there without one having to ask for it" and to show "dependence, a feeling of a need for rescue" and to test continually limits and boundaries.

# Your Amazing Newborn Baby

## It is astonishing what a baby can do within minutes of his or her birth.

In 1992, Dr. Lennart Righard, a Swedish obstetrician, videoed newborns who had been placed on their mothers' abdomens, showing that the supposedly helpless babies could inch very slowly upward, without any help, towards their mother's breast and suckle when they arrived there. They can grasp a finger, most can breathe unaided within minutes, and can cry surprisingly loudly, without shedding tears, to communicate their needs.

### REACTING TO NEW SURROUNDINGS

Newborns also seem to arrive pre-programmed to like human faces. Research (see Medical Reference List, p. 152) shows they follow a facelike pattern with more interest than other similar colourful patterns, and can see their mothers' faces well—focusing best at about 30 cm (12 inches), the distance between the baby's eyes and the mother's when the baby is being held to the breast. They are able to follow a moving object with their eyes, and turn towards lights. However, newborn babies' eye movements are often not well coordinated at first, and may sometimes move independently of each other, producing a slight squint which usually resolves itself on its own. They won't like bright delivery-room lights either, because the most they may have experienced so far has been in the form of an orange glow diffused by the mother's abdomen (if, for instance, the mother was sunbathing and had her tummy exposed).

A newborn baby will also recognize his or her mother's voice right away, as this is the one that could be heard the most clearly in the womb, as it reverberated through her body. In fact, according to research carried out in Chicago in 1975, newborn babies respond far better to female voices in general, although all voices heard in the outside world will sound rather different from the tones the baby was used to in the womb, muffled as they were for months by layers of muscle, fat and amniotic fluid. As soon as they are born, babies can even "walk" if held firmly under the arms with their feet on a flat surface. They will turn to and prefer the smell of milk over that of other substances, and, according to Harvard University paediatrician Dr. Berry Brazelton, they will show, by changes in their suckling rate, that they can tell the difference between human milk and formula milk. Within a few days, your baby will recognize your smell, voice and appearance, and the taste of your breast milk, as no two milks have exactly the same composition or scent.

## HAVING TO ADJUST TO THIS NEW LIFE

Within seconds of birth, a newborn is already making massive adjustments to life outside the womb. These may not be obvious, yet they are still major achievements. They include getting used

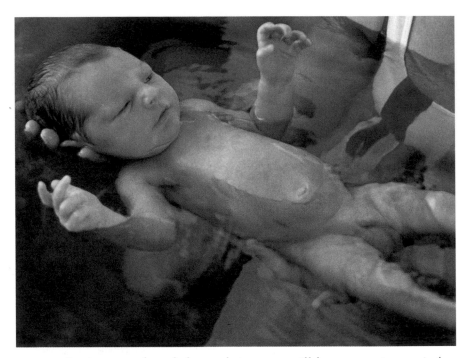

*ABOVE: Resting a newborn baby gently in water will be a reassuring reminder of his or her previous life in the womb.*

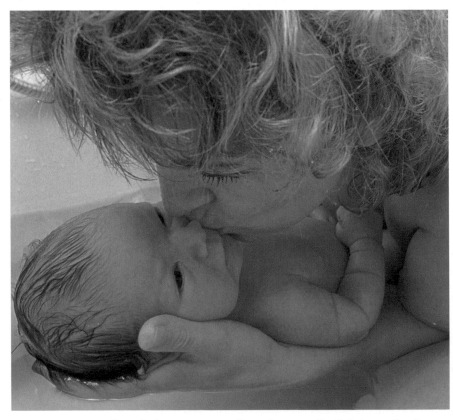

*ABOVE: Newborn babies recognize the unique smell of their mothers' skin over that of a stranger within hours of delivery.*

to no longer having a buoyant liquid environment, as well as to the initially alarming freedom of having no confinements after being curled up in an increasingly cramped, cushioned space for so long. Newborns breathe air for the first time, after having had oxygen piped to them in the placenta's blood supply. (Dr. Leboyer suggests that the first breaths may sting airways which before only knew fluid, like "the first cigarette or first whisky burns your throat".) Being cold is another new experience, and an unpleasant shock (remember that the average room temperature is a lot cooler than it is inside you). Babies arrive sopping wet, and because of the high surface-to-body weight ratio, lose heat fast. Their homoeostatic (temperature-maintaining) mechanism is not yet mature, so they need warm, soft, loose wrappings and a cuddle from their parents—and quick.

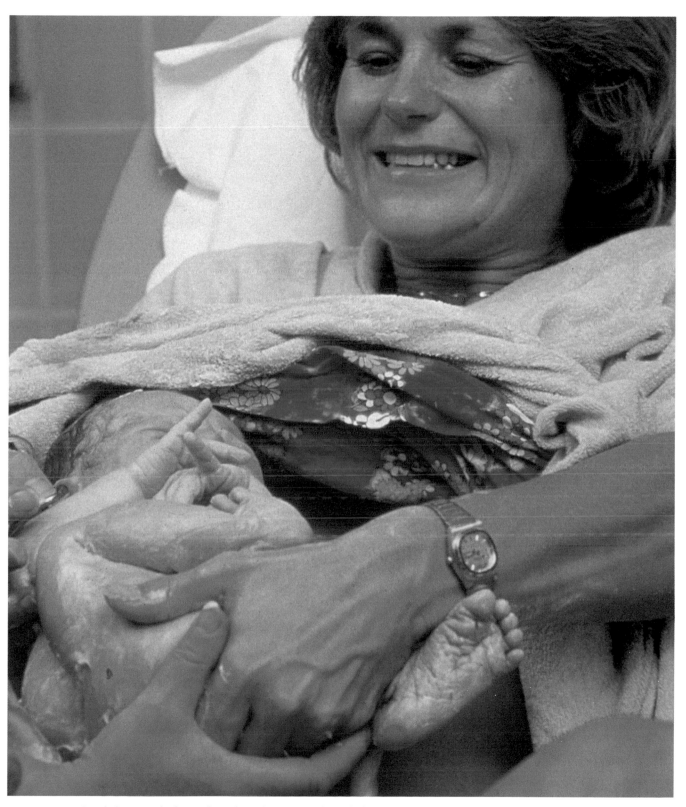

*ABOVE: Swedish research shows that if you leave a newborn baby resting on his or her mother's tummy, the baby will, given time, manage to inch towards her breast, the place where he or she instinctively knows her milk is.*

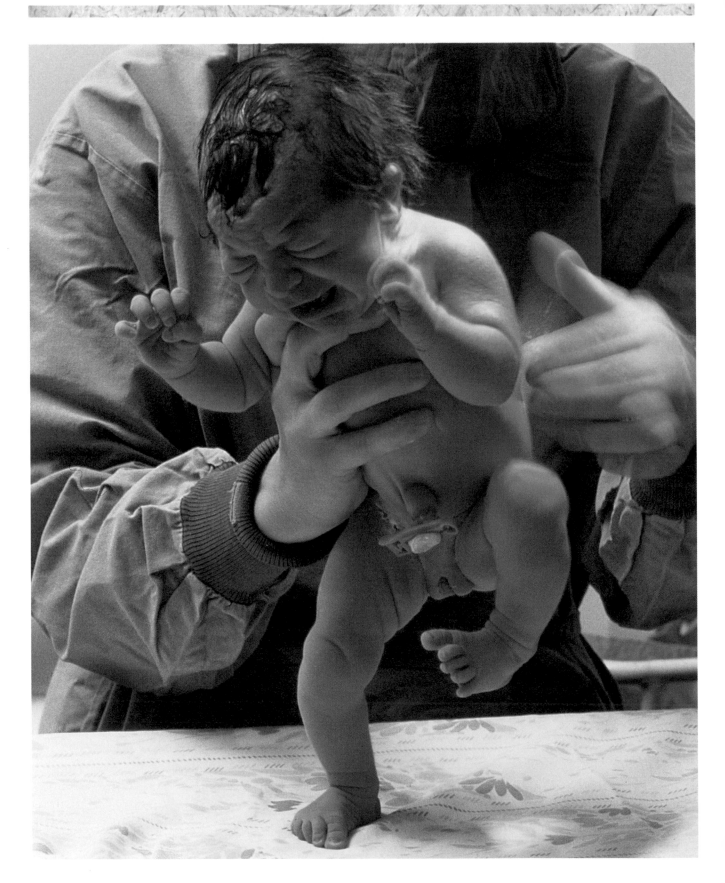

## BONDING

From the moment of birth, a baby is also powerfully primed to bond with his or her mother. Mothers themselves often say seeing and holding their baby for the first time was literally like falling in love at first sight; others report they didn't feel much at first, but their attachment to their new baby grew with time; many described it as more like a recognition of someone beloved whom they already knew. "There was nothing romantic or solemn about it. No obligations, no fancy games. We'd met. Just that. Somewhere in the spirit, we were friends." (Leslie Kenton, *All I Ever Wanted Was a Baby*.)

The warmth and feel of your presence will comfort and reassure your baby more than anything, as the confines of your body have been his or her entire world up until a few minutes ago, and now you are needed for shelter and continuity in the new one. If you breast-feed as soon as you can, the action of suckling on your nipples, perhaps extracting a little colostrum (the clear, immensely nourishing pre-milk) and nuzzling into your breast, will let the baby know he or she is, after the hard physical work and trauma of birth, safe at last, welcome and loved.

However, bonding is not just a psychological phenomenon; both you and your baby get a great boost of hormonal help, too. Between 1 and 12 hours after birth both the mother and child have high levels of beta-endorphin hormones, which

*LEFT: Newly delivered babies can, if you hold them upright and place their feet on a flat surface, appear to walk. They lose this reflex after about six weeks, however.*

### YOUR BABY'S APGAR SCORE

The Apgar scoring system is used to assess babies' well-being just after birth. Five different factors are considered and each is allocated between 0 and 2 points, up to a maximum of ten points overall. You probably will not notice the Apgar checks being carried out, as it is usually more a matter of a nurse, obstetrician or midwife running an experienced eye over your baby.

| Factors | Score | | |
|---|---|---|---|
| | 0 | 1 | 2 |
| Heart rate | Absent | slow ( <100 bpm ) | >100 bpm |
| Respiratory effort | Absent | slow, irregular | good, crying |
| Muscle tone | Flaccid | some limb flexion | active motion |
| Reflex ability | No response | cry | vigorous cry |
| Colour | Blue, or pale | body pink, limbs blue | completely pink* |

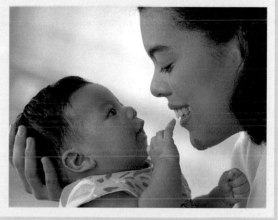

* Dark-skinned babies tend to be a purplish-grey when born. Their Apgar scores will be assessed by an examination of the soles of their feet, their fingernails and the area around their mouth.

(From *Evaluation of the Newborn* by Hill & Stephenson, in *Turnbull's Obstetrics*, 1995, pub. Churchill Livingstone)

produce a natural high, and greatly enhance the baby's learning ability. You both also have high levels of the milk-releasing hormone prolactin, which triggers instinctive behaviour—what's described as "staying at home, nurturing behaviour" for you, and nipple-searching and nuzzling behaviour in your baby. Beta-endorphins have another practical function, too, deadening any residual pain or discomfort either you or your baby may feel immediately after childbirth. The hormone oxytocin, which encouraged your womb to contract during labour and triggers the release

of colostrum and milk from your breasts, also promotes amnesia. This helps memories of any troubling aspects of the birth to recede, leaving you freer and less distracted to discover and explore each other in peace.

### YOUR BABY'S APGAR SCORE

Babies are assessed one to five minutes after birth. The Apgar scoring system (named after Dr. Virginia Apgar) is usually used to check their well-being, through their heart rate, breathing, muscle tone, reflex responses and skin colour, with each factor allocated 0 to 2 points.

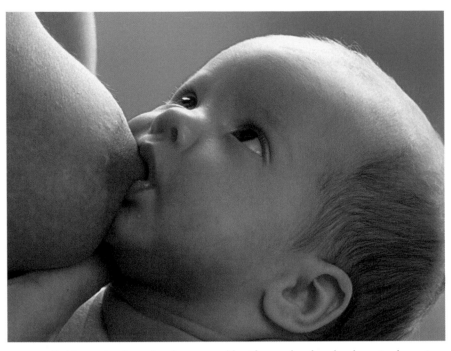

*ABOVE: Babies arrive knowing how to suckle. If a mother brushes her nipple against her baby's cheek, the child will turn towards it and open its lips.*

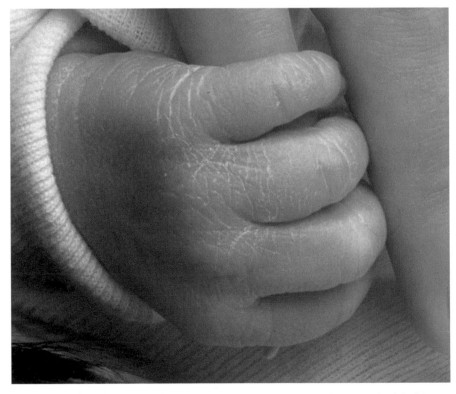

*ABOVE: The grip of newborns is surprisingly powerful, and they find holding on to one of your fingers very reassuring. Mothers often instinctively let their new baby hold one of their fingers while they are breast- or bottle-feeding.*

A baby scoring 7+ at one minute is judged to be doing fine. A baby scoring between 4 and 7 would be monitored carefully and rechecked at regular intervals, and given treatment or help as necessary. A newborn scoring below 4 would need resuscitation. The latter involves extracting any mucus from the airways with a catheter, then giving the baby oxygen.

### BREATHING

Babies usually show regular, rhythmical breathing of 30 to 50 times a minute within the first few minutes. Initial irregular breathing can fluctuate between 15 and 100 breaths a minute until babies hit their stride. They can usually get about 70 per cent of their breathing capacity working within their first few gasps.

### SKIN COLOUR

When born, Caucasian babies are usually a dull red/dull bluish-grey—dark-skinned babies are a purplish-grey—covered in waxy vernix. It is not unusual for newborns to appear mottled at first, or for their skin to turn red from head to foot if they are crying furiously. Occasionally in the first couple of days you might see what is called the Harlequin Change, where just one side of the body flushes, with a midline down the centre. Don't worry about any of these. It is just your baby's immature circulation settling down. Skin colour will be uniformly normal, except for bluish hands and feet when cold, within about 48 hours.

### REFLEXES

There are 73 reflexes present in a newborn baby that can be tested, but doctors only routinely use about half a dozen to assess how the baby is, and to exclude the possibility of major neurological problems. The reflexes they check include:

### Grasp Reflex

Your baby's small hand tightens firmly over your finger when you slide it into his or her palm, and will grip harder if you try to remove it. This reflex develops after only 12 weeks in the womb.

### Traction Response

When you gently pull babies up into a sitting position by their hands, they flex their elbows. This reflex develops about three weeks before the birth.

### Moro Reflex

This is essentially the baby's response to being made to feel suddenly insecure. The child is held on his or her back in the nurse's, midwife's or obstetrician's hands, head supported. The head is allowed to drop back abruptly a little, and the child responds by flinging out his or her arms and extending the legs and head. Not surprisingly, this is, according to the standard medical textbooks "usually accompanied by crying". Another basic reflex tested, called the startle reflex, produces a similar reaction, but the stimulus is not a sudden loss of security in space, but a loud noise, or a tap on the baby's chest.

### Stepping or Walking Reflex

If you hold your newborn baby under his or her arms and place the feet on a flat surface, he or she will make stepping movements, as if walking, although often one leg gets caught up behind the other. Babies

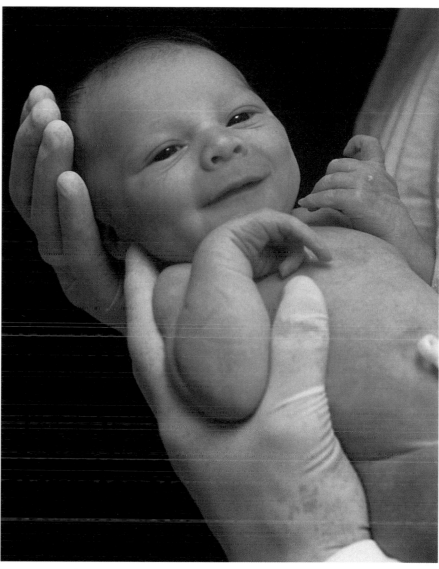

ABOVE: *Babies are not "supposed" to smile until they are about six weeks old, but parents report social smiles (made in response to a smile from them) rather than smiles when content, from two weeks; but most sceptical professionals say it's "just wind".*

can do this until they are about five or six weeks old, when they lose the knack. Most do not try supported walking again until they are five to seven months old, when parents will find themselves constantly holding stepping toddlers upright as they walk up and down, delighted with their new skill. Less mature babies can "walk", too, but will do so on their toes.

### Rooting Reflex

Rooting is the search-for-milk reflex all normal, full-term babies have at birth, and they will, given the chance, prove it by suckling from you within minutes of their arrival. This is an automatic response that takes place when a baby's cheek comes into contact with the mother's breast or nipple. Brushing the corner of babies' mouths with a nipple causes them to open their mouths, pout their lips and move their tongues.

### Asymmetric Tonic Neck Reflex

In this reflex, if a baby is lying with his or her head turned to one side, the arm or leg on that side will extend while the other remains flexed.

### Latching on, Sucking on, Suckling and Swallowing

All these terms describe a reflexive behaviour. ("Latching on" means the way babies place their mouths on the nipple of a breast or bottle to suck from it.) They do, however, involve a surprisingly complex coordinated pattern of feeding movements for the lips, tongue, palate and throat. This entire reflex system developed by the time your baby was 32 weeks old in your womb, although he or she only became strong enough for feeding by 36 weeks. (This is why immature babies born before 36 weeks need feeding help.)

Some of these reflexes and abilities, such as suckling, seeing their mothers' faces at 30cm (12 inches) away and rooting, are exactly what babies need for survival; others, such as the stepping reflex, are the fore-runners of skills they will not need until later. Yet, your baby has made the astonishing transition from inhabiting someone else's body—yours—to living as a separate being. Although still closely connected and dependent upon you, your tiny son or daughter is now fully equipped to be a part of the outside world, and with your love and care your baby will grow strong and flourish faster than you had ever imagined.

# Medical Reference List

The following bibliography lists the references from clinical journals, books and research theses which support the text in the different chapters. We list journal names, article titles, page numbers and volume references. We also list publishers, publication dates and authors, for all references, in case readers would like to follow them up more fully.

## NATURAL GENDER SELECTION

James, W. H., *Human Biology*, "The Human Sex Ratio", Parts 1 & 2 (1987)

Little, B. B. et al., *Aviation Space Environmental Medicine*, "Pilot and Astronaut Offspring: Possible G-Force Effects on Human Sex Ratio", vol. 58, pp. 77–79 (1987)

Lloyd, M. and Lyster, W. R., *Journal of the Royal College of Physicians*, "Low Sex Ratios in Children of Men with Alcohol-Related Occupations", vol. 222, pp. 280–281 (1987)

Lloyd, Dr. Melody (Ninewells Hospital Medical School, Dundee), *British Medical Journal*, "Slugs and Snails Against Sugar and Spice", pp. 24–31 (December 1988)

Papa, François and Labro, Françoise, *Boy or Girl?* (Souvenir Press, 1984)

Teitelbaum, M. S., *The Journal of Biosocial Science*, "Factors Affecting Sex Ratio in Large Populations", vol. 2, pp. 61–71 (1970)

## THE DEVELOPMENT OF YOUR BABY IN THE WOMB

Boué, André, *Foetal Medicine—Perinatal Diagnosis & Management* (Oxford University Press, 1995)

Chamberlain, Professor G., ed., *Turnbull's Obstetrics* (Churchill Livingstone, Edinburgh, 1995)

Clements, Michelle, *The Pre- and Perinatal Psychology Journal* *, "Observation on Certain Aspects of Foetal Behavior in Response to Auditory Stimuli", vol. 6, pp. 217–235, (1977)

Creasy & Resnick, *Maternal and Foetal Medicine* (W. B. Saunders, 1994)

DeSnoo, K., *Monatsschrift fur Gubertschilfe & Gynaekologie*, "Das Trinkebuds Kind im Uterus", vol. 105, pp. 88–97 (1937)

England, Professor Marjorie, *A Colour Atlas of Life Before Birth* (Wolfe Medical Publications, 1993)

Gellrich, Dr. M., *Prenatal Perception, Learning and Bonding*, "Development of Music Before Birth and in Early Childhood" (Blum, T., ed., Leonardo, Hong Kong, 1993)

Johnstone, Peter G. B., *The Newborn Child*, 7th ed. (Churchill Livingstone, Edinburgh, 1994)

Sharp, Professor F., ed., *Foetal Growth* (Royal College of Obstetrics & Gynaecology, 20th study group, 1989)

Spencer, J. A. D. and Wood, R. H. T., eds., *Intrapartum Foetal Surveillance* (Royal College of Obstetrics & Gynaecology Press, 1993)

Tatzer, E. et al., *Early Human Development*, "Discrimination of Taste and Preference for Sweetness etc.: Fetus Reacting to Sweet/Bitter Taste", vol. 12, pp. 23–30

Thorburn & Hardy, eds., *Textbook of Foetal Physiology* (Oxford Medical Publishing, 1994)

Whitehead, Andrews, and Chamberlain, Professor G., "Characterization of Nausea and Vomiting in Early Pregnancy: a Survey of 1,000 Women" (Department of Obstetrics & Gynaecology, St. George's Hospital, 1976)

## MOVEMENT—WHAT DO BABIES DO IN THERE?

De Vries, J. I. P., *Early Human Development*, "The Emergence of Fetal Behavior", vol. 12 (1985)

*Early Human Development*, vol. 7, pp. 301–322 (1982)/vol. 12, pp. 99–102 (1993)/vol. 25, pp. 85–144 (1996) (Elsevier Press, USA)

Sival, D. A., *Early Human Development*, "Studies in Fetal Motor Behavior", vol. 34 (1991)

## CHECKING YOUR BABY'S WELL-BEING IN THE WOMB

Bewley, S. et al., *British Journal of Obstetrics and Gynaecology*, "First Trimester Measurements of Foetal Nuchal Translucency etc.", vol. 102, pp. 386–388 (1995)

Chamberlain, Professor G., *Turnbull's Obstetrics*, "Prenatal Diagnosis" (Churchill Livingstone, Edinburgh, 1995)

*Current Opinions in Obstetrics and Gynaecology*, "Prenatal Diagnosis of Major Congenital Malformations", vol. 6, pp. 459–467 (1994)

Firth, Boyd et al., *The Lancet*, "Severe Limb Abnormalities After Chorionic Villus Sampling", vol. 337, pp. 762–763 (1991)

Johnson, Jo-Ann M. et al., *Fetal Diagnosis and Therapy*, "Early Amniocentesis Study: A Randomized Clinical Trial of Early vs. Midtrimester Amniocentesis", vol. 11, pp. 85–93 (1996)

Medical Research Council Working Party on the Evaluation of Chorionic Villus Sampling, *The Lancet*, "MRC European Trial of Chorionic Villus Sampling", vol. 337, pp. 1491–1493 (1991)

Nicholaides, Professor Kypros, *The Lancet*, "Comparison of CVS and Amniocentesis of Foetal Karotyping at 10 to 13 Weeks' Gestation", vol. 344, pp. 435–439 (1994)

Parry, Vivienne, *The Antenatal Testing Handbook* (Pan Books, 1994)

Rodeck, Charles H. and Johnson, Pam, *Turnbull's Obstetrics*, "Prenatal Diagnosis" (Churchill Livingstone, Edinburgh, 1995)

Royal College of Obstetrics & Gynaecology, *Guidance on Ultrasound Practices in Early Pregnancy* (1995)

Wexler, Keith and Laurie, *The ABCs of Prenatal Diagnosis* (ed. by Professor Paul Wexler; Genassist, USA, 1994)

## UNBORN BABIES' REACTIONS TO THE TESTS

*AIMS Quarterly Journal*, "Jumping Babies", vol. 5/7, pp. 15–17

Baker, R. A., *Obstetrics and Gynaecology Journal*, "Technologic Intervention in Obstetrics", vol. 2, p. 51 (1978)

Birlholz, J. and Stephens, J. C., *American Journal of Roentology*, "Fetal Movement Patterns: A Possible Means of Defining Neurological Development Milestones *In Utero*", vol. 130, pp. 537–540

Chamberlain, Dr. David B., *The International Journal of Pre- and Perinatal Psychology and Medicine*, "The Sentient Prenate: What Every Parent Should Know", pp. 9–31 (Fall 1994)

Chamberlain, Dr. David B., *The International Journal of Pre- and Perinatal Psychology and Medicine*, "What Babies Are Teaching Us About Violence", pp. 57–74 (Winter 1995)

Emerson, Dr. William, *The International Journal of Pre- and Perinatal Psychology and Medicine*, "The Vulnerable Prenate", pp. 125–142 (1996)

Hill, L. M. et al., *American Journal of Obstetrics and Gynecology*, "Immediate After-effects of Amniocentesis on Fetal Breathing and Gross Body Movement", vol. 135, pp. 689–690

Manning, F. A., Platt, L. D. et al., *British Medical Journal*, "Effect of Amniocentesis on Foetal Breathing Movements", vol. 2, pp. 1582–1583 (1977)

Ron, M. and Polishuk, W. Z., *British Journal of Obstetrics and Gynaecology*, "The Response of Foetal Heartrate to Amniocentesis", vol. 83, p. 768 (1976)

**DOES YOUR UNBORN BABY FEEL YOUR EMOTIONS?**
Bunstan, M. N. and Coker, A. L., *American Journal of Public Health*, "Maternal Attitude Toward Pregnancy and the Risk of Neonatal Death", vol. 84/3, pp. 411–414 (1994)

Carey, W. B., *Clinical Paediatrics*, "Maternal Anxiety and Infantile Colic: is There a Relationship?", vol. 7, pp. 188–194 (1968)

Carlson, B. and LaBarba, R. C., *The International Journal of Behavioral Development*, "Maternal Emotionality During Pregnancy and Reproductive Outcome", vol. 2, pp. 343–376

Cheek, Dr. David, *The International Journal of Pre- and Perinatal Psychology and Medicine*, "Are Telepathy, Clairvoyance and 'Hearing' Possible *in Utero*? Suggestive Evidence as Revealed During Hypnotic Age-Regression Studies of Prenatal Memory", vol. 7/2, pp. 125–137 (Winter 1992)

Correia, I. B., *The Impact of Television Stimuli on the Prenatal Infant* (doctoral dissertation, University of South Wales, Sydney, Australia)

David, H. P., Drytrych, Z., and Matejcek, Z. et al., *Born Unwanted: Developmental Effects of Denied Abortion* (Czechoslovak Medical Press, Prague, 1988)

Ellis, Lee and Peckham, William, *The International Journal of Pre- and Perinatal Psychology and Medicine*, "Prenatal Stress and Handedness Among Offspring", pp. 135–143 (Winter 1991)

Farber, E. A. et al., *Early Human Development*, "The Relationship of Prenatal Maternal Anxiety to Infant Behavior and Mother-Infant Interactions During the First Six Months of Life", vol. 5, pp. 267–277

Hepper, Professor Peter (Queen's University, Belfast), *The Links Between Maternal Anxiety and Foetal Behaviour* (Report of the Biennial Meeting of the Marcé Society, London, Sept. 1996)

Illingworth, Ronald, ed., *Development of the Infant and Young Child*, "Pre- and Perinatal Factors", pp. 25–26, 251 (Marcé Society)

*International Journal of Behavioral Development*, "Maternal Emotionality During Pregnancy and Reproductive Outcome: a Review of the Literature", vol. 2, pp. 343–376

Joffe, J. M., *Studies on the Development and Behavior of the Nervous System*, "Hormonal Mediation of the Effects of Prenatal Stress on Offspring Behavior" (*Early Influences*, vol. 4, Gottlieb, G., ed.), pp. 107–144 (Academic Press, New York, 1978)

Lou, Professor Hans, *Prenatal Stressors for the Mother Affect Foetal Brain Development* (John F. Kennedy Institute, Glostrup, Denmark, Biannual Meeting of the Marcé Society, London, Sept. 1996)

Olds, C., *The International Journal of Pre- and Perinatal Psychology and Medicine*, "A Sound Start in Life", vol. 1/1, pp. 82–85 (1986)

Pert, Candace, *Cybernetics*, "Neuropeptide Receptors and Emotions", vol. 1/4, pp. 33–34

Rossi, N. et al., *The International Journal of Pre- and Perinatal Psychology and Medicine*, "Maternal Stress and Fetal Motor Behavior: A Preliminary Report", vol. 3/4, pp. 311–318 (1989)

Sontag, L. W., *The American Journal of Obstetrics and Gynecology*, "The Significance of Fetal Environmental Differences", vol. 42, pp. 996–1003 (1941)

Van den Bergh, B. R. H., *The International Journal of Pre- and Perinatal Psychology and Medicine*, "The Influence of Maternal Emotions During Pregnancy on Fetal and Neonatal Behavior" (Winter 1990)

Van den Bergh, B. R. H., "Maternal Emotions During Pregnancy", Zimmer et al. (1982)

Verny, Thomas, with Kelly, John, *The Secret Life of the Unborn Child*, pp. 57–9 (Summit Books, 1981; Sphere Books, 1982; reprinted Warner Books, 1993)

War, A. J., *Child Psychiatry and Human Development*, "Stress and Childhood Psychopathology", vol. 22/2, pp. 97–110 (1991)

**WHAT YOUR UNBORN BABY CAN LEARN**
Chamberlain, Dr. David B., *Life in the Womb: Dangers and Opportunities* (International Congress Aprendizaje y Comunicacion Pre y Postnatal, Valencia, Spain, June 1996)

DeCasper, A. et al., *Infant Behaviour and Development* "Foetal Reactions to Recurrent Maternal Speech", vol.17/2, pp. 159–164

Diamond, M. C., *Enriching Heredity* (The Free Press, New York, 1989)

Logan, Brent, *The International Journal of Pre- and Perinatal Psychology and Medicine*, "Infant Outcomes of a Prenatal Stimulation Pilot Study", pp. 7–31 (Fall 1991)

Manrique, B. et al., *Prenatal Perception, Learning and Bonding*, "Nurturing Parents to Stimulate Their Children from Prenatal Stage to Three

Years of Age" (Blum, T., ed., Berlin and Hong Kong, Leonardo, 1993)

Nakae, K., *Japanese Journal of Education Research*, "A Historical Study on the Thought of *Taikyo*", vol. 50, pp. 343–352 (1983)

Panthuraamphorn, Dr. Chairat, *Prenatal Perception, Learning, and Bonding*, "Prenatal Infant Stimulation Program" (Blum, T., ed., Berlin and Hong Kong, Leonardo, 1993)

Van de Carr, R., et al., *Prenatal and Perinatal Psychology and Medicine: A Comprehensive Survey of Research and Practice*, "Effects of a Prenatal Intervention Program" (Feydor-Freyburgh, P. and Vogel, M. L., eds., Parthenon Publishing, 1988)

Van de Carr, F. René and Lehrer, Marc, *The Prenatal Classroom—a Parent's Guide to Teaching Your Baby in the Womb* (Humanics Learning, Atlanta, Georgia, 1992)

Wittrock, M. C., *The Brain and Psychology* (Academic Press, New York, 1980)

**SEXUALITY DURING PREGNANCY— WHAT YOUR BABY MAY NOTICE**
Chamberlain, Dr. David B., *The International Journal of Pre- and Perinatal Psychology and Medicine*, "Is There Intelligence Before Birth?", pp. 217–236 (Spring 1992)

Chayen, B., Tejania, N., Verma, U. L. et al., *Acta Obstetrica Gynecologica Scandinavica*, "Foetal Heartrate Changes and Uterine Activity During Coitus", vol. 65, pp. 853–855 (1986)

Godlin, R. C. et al., *Obstetrics and Gynaecology*, "Uterine Tension and Foetal Heartrate During Maternal Orgasm", vol. 39/1, pp. 125–127 (1972)

Shirozu, Hiroaki et al., *Early Human Development*, "Penile Tumescence in the Human Foetus at Full Term A Preliminary Report", vol. 41, pp. 159–166 (1995)

**WHAT YOUR BABY CAN HEAR IN THE WOMB**
Birnholz, J. C. and Benacerraf, B. R., *Science*, "The Development of Human Foetal Hearing", vol. 222, pp. 516–518 (1983)

Busnel, M. C. et al., *Annals of New York Academy of Sciences*, "Fetal Audition", vol. 662, pp. 118–134 (1992)

Hepper, Professor Peter, *Foetal Psychology: An Embryonic Science*, "Foetal Behaviour", pp. 131–149 (Queen's University, Belfast)

Johnson, R. L. et al., *The Journal of Reproductive Medicine*, "Foetal Acoustic Stimulation as an Adjunct to External Cephalic Version", vol. 40, pp. 696–698 (1995)

Liley, Albert, T*he Australian and New Zealand Journal of Psychiatry*, "The Foetus as a Personality", vol. 6/99 (1972)

Querleu, Denis et al., *Seminars in Perinatology*, "Hearing by the Human Foetus?", vol. 13, pp. 409–420 (Department of Obstetrics and Gynaecology, Pavilion Paul Gelle Roubaix and University of Lille, France, 1989)

Read, J. and Miller, F., *The American Journal of Obstetrics and Gynecology*, "Fetal Heartrate Acceleration in Response to Acoustic Stimulation as a Measure of Fetal of Well-Being", vol. 129, pp. 512–539 (1977)

Truby, Henry, *Child Language*, "Prenatal and Neonatal Speech, Pre-speech and Infantile Speech Lexicon" (1975, special ed. of *Word* 27, parts 1–3)

Van de Carr, F. René and Lehrer, Marc, *The Prenatal Classroom—a Parent's Guide to Teaching Your Baby in the Womb* (Humanics Learning, Atlanta, Georgia, 1992)

Zimmer et al., *Early Human Development*, "Response of the Premature Foetus to Stimulation by Speech Sounds", vol. 33, pp. 207–215 (1993)

THE DREAMS OF PREGNANT WOMEN AND THEIR UNBORN BABIES
Birnholz, J. and Stephens, J. C. et al., *Science*, "The Development of Human Foetal Eye Movement Patterns", vol. 213, pp. 679–681

Emerson, Dr. William, *Infant and Childbirth Re-facilitation* (Human Potential Resources, Petaluma, USA, 1984)

Laing, R. D., *The Facts of Life* (Allen Lane, 1976)

Parkes, M. J., *The Foetal and Neonatal Brain Stem* (Cambridge University Press, 1991)

*Primitive Study IV: Child Development*, "Neonatal Smiling in REM States", vol. 42, pp. 1657–1661

Rank, Otto, *The Trauma of Birth* (Warner Torch Books, New York, 1934)

Ridgeway, Roy, *The Unborn Child: How to Recognize and Overcome Prenatal Trauma* (Wildwood House, 1987)

Stukane, Eileen, *The Dream World of Pregnancy* (Airlift Books, UK, 1995)

Vaughan, Christopher, *How Life Begins—The Science of the Womb* (Times Books USA, 1996)

Verny, Thomas, with Kelly, John, *The Secret Life of the Unborn Child* (Summit Books, 1981; Sphere Books, 1982; reprinted Warner Books, 1993)

TWINS AND YOU
Barron, D. S., *Health*, "Once There Were Two", pp. 84–90 (Sept. 1996)

Emerson, Dr. William, *The International Journal of Pre- and Perinatal Psychology and Medicine*,

"The Vulnerable Prenate", pp. 125–142 (Spring 1996)

Gallaher, M. W., Costigan, K., and Johnson, T. R. (Department of Obstetrics and Gynecology, Johns Hopkins University School of Medicine, Baltimore), *American Journal of Obstetrics and Gynecology*, "Fetal Heart Rate Accelerations, Fetal Movements and Fetal Behavior Patterns in Twin Gestations", vol. 167, pp. 1140–1144 (1992)

Noble, Elisabeth, *The International Journal of Prenatal and Perinatal Studies*, "Resolution of Habitual Abortion in the Survivor of a 'Vanishing Twin' Pregnancy", vol. 1/1, pp. 117–120 (1991)

Piontelli, Alessandra, *The International Journal of Psychoanalysis*, "Infant Observations from Before Birth", vol. 68, p. 453 (1987)

GAMES YOUR UNBORN BABY PLAYS
Freeman, M., *The International Journal of Pre- and Perinatal Psychology and Medicine*, "Is Infant Learning Egocentric or Duocentric? Was Piaget Wrong?", vol. 2/1, pp. 25–42 (1987)

Piontelli, Alessandra, *The International Journal of Psychoanalysis*, "Infant Observations from Before Birth", vol. 68, p. 453 (1987)

Straub, Mary F., *The International Journal of Pre- and Perinatal Psychology and Medicine*, "A Theory of the Psychological Consequences of Umbilical Cord Manipulation by the Fetus", vol. 7/1, (Fall 1992)

Van de Carr, René F and Lehrer, Marc, *The Prenatal Classroom*, Curriculum section (Humanics Learning, Atlanta, Georgia, 1992)

CAN PREBORNS AND NEWBORNS FEEL PAIN?
*Birth*, "Letters", pp. 124–125 (June 1986)

Chamberlain, Dr. David B., *Babies Remember Birth* (Chapter 7, Ballantine Books, 1990)

Chamberlain, Dr. David B., in *Cyborg Babies: From Techno-Sex to Techno-Tots* (Davies-Fflod, Robbe and Dumit, James, eds., Routledge, London, 1997)

"Foetal Sentience", All-Party Parliamentary Pro-Life Group (UK, Aug. 1996)

Fisk, Nicholas et al., work conducted by Queen Charlotte's Hospital, UK, 1985

Grunau, R. V. E. and Craig, K. D., *Pain*, "Pain Expressions in Neonates: Facial Action and Cry", vol. 28, pp. 341–395 (1987)

McGraw, Myrtle, *Child Development*, "Neural Maturation as Exemplified in the Changing Reactions to the Infant Pin Prick", vol. 12/1, pp. 31–42 (1941)

Paintin, D., "Can a Foetus Feel Pain?" (comments on "Foetal Sentience" paper, *above*, St. Mary's Hospital, London, 1996)

Sherman et al., *Journal of Comparative Psychology*, "Sensory-Motor Responses in Infants", vol. 5, pp. 53–68 (1925)

Talbert et al., *Obstetrics and Gynaecology*, "Adrenal Corticol Response to Circumcision in the Neonate", vol. 48, pp. 208-210 (1975)

Williamson, Paul and Marvel, *Paediatrics*, "Physiologic Stress Reduction by a Local Anaesthetic During Newborn Circumcision", vol. 71/1, pp. 36–40 (1983)

NOISES YOUR BABY MAKES IN THE WOMB
Freed, F., *The American Journal of Obstetrics and Gynecology*, "Report of a Case of Vaginitus Uterinus", vol. 14, pp. 87–89 (1927)

Ryder, G. H., *The American Journal of Obstetrics and Gynecology*, "Vaginitus Uterinus", vol. 46, pp. 867–872 (1943)

Thiery et al., *Journal of Obstetrics and Gynaecology of the British Commonwealth*, "Vaginitus Uterinus", vol. 80, pp. 183–185 (1973)

PREPARING YOUR BABY FOR BIRTH
Balaskas, Janet and Gordon, Yehudi, *Water Birth* (Thorsons, UK, 1992)

Lake, Frank, *Constricted Confusion: Exploration of a Pre- and Perinatal Paradigm* (published privately)

Leboyer, Frederick, *Birth Without Violence* (Knopf, 1996)

Panthuraamphorn, Dr. Chairat (Hua Chiew General Hospital, Bangkok), *The International Journal of Pre- and Perinatal Psychology and Medicine* "How to Maximize Human Potential at Birth", pp. 117–126 (Winter 1994)

OVERDUE BABIES
Cardazo, Professor Linda, *Turnbull's Obstetrics*, "Prolonged Pregnancy" chapter (Churchill Livingstone, Edinburgh, 1995)

Chalmers, Ian, *Benefits and Hazards of the New Obstetrics*, "Intervention… in Obstetric Practice" (Chard and Richards, eds., Spastics International Medical Publications, London, 1977)

Studd, John, ed., *Progress in Obstetrics and Gynaecology*, "Placental Pathology" section, vol. 3 (Churchill Livingstone, Edinburgh, 1983)

MEMORIES OF BEING IN THE WOMB—AND BEING BORN
Chamberlain, Dr. David B., *The International Journal of Pre- and Perinatal Psychology and Medicine*, "The Significance of Birth Memories", vol. 2/4, pp. 136–154 (Summer 1988)

Chamberlain, Dr. David B., *The Journal of the American Academy of Medical Hypnoanalysts*, "Reliability of Birth Memory: Observations from Mother and Child Pairs in Hypnosis", pp. 89–98 (Dec. 1986)

Cheek, David B., *The American Journal of Clinical Hypnosis*, "Maladjustment Patterns Apparently Related to Imprinting at Birth", vol. 18, pp. 75–82 (1975)

Cheek, David B., *The International Journal of Pre- and Perinatal Psychology and Medicine*, "Prenatal and Perinatal Imprints: Apparent Prenatal Consciousness as Revealed by Hypnosis", vol. 1/2, pp. 97–110 (1986)

Emerson, Dr. William, *Infant and Child Birth Re-facilitation* (Human Potential Resources, Petaluma, USA, 1984)

Emerson, Dr. William, *Life, Birth and Rebirth: The Hazy Mirrors* (Self and Society, July 1978)

Fodor, N., *Search for the Beloved: a Clinical Investigation of the Trauma of Birth and Prenatal Cognition* (Hermitage Press, New York, 1949)

Kelsey, D. E. R., *Journal of the Mental Sciences/British Journal of Psychiatry*, "Fantasies of Birth and Prenatal Experience Recovered from Patients Undergoing Hypnoanalysis", vol. 99, pp. 216–233 (1953)

Laibow, R. E., *The International Journal of Pre- and Perinatal Psychology and Medicine*, "Birth Recall: a Clinical Report", vol. 1/1, pp. 78–81 (1986)

Mathison, L. A., *Mothering*, "Does Your Child Remember?", vol. 21, pp. 103–107 (1981)

Pribam, Karl, *The American Psychologist*, "The Cognitive Revolution and Mind/Brain Issues", vol. 41/5, pp. 507–520 (1986)

Raikov, Vladimir, *American Journal of Clinical Hypnosis*, "Age Regression to Infancy by Adult Subjects in Deep Hypnosis", vol. 22, pp. 156–163 (1980)

Rank, Otto, *The Trauma of Birth* (Harcourt and Brace, New York, 1929)

Ridgeway, Roy, *The Unborn Child: How to Recognize and Overcome Prenatal Trauma* (Wildwood Press, 1987)

## LABOUR—WHAT TO EXPECT
Bradford, Nikki and Chamberlain, Professor Geoffrey, *Pain Relief in Labour*, incl. section on "Acupuncture in Childbirth" (HarperCollins, UK, 1995)

Chamberlain, Dr. David B., *The International Journal of Pre- and Perinatal Psychology and Medicine*, "What Babies Are Teaching Us About Violence", pp. 117–126 (Winter 1995)

Leboyer, Frederick, *Birth Without Violence* (Knopf, 1996)

*Midwives Chronicle*, "Anaesthesia and Analgesia" (Queen Mother's Hospital, Yorkhill, Glasgow, 1975)

*The National Birthday Trust Survey on Pain Relief in Labour* (1993)

*The Nursing Times*, "Aromatherapy" (March 1994, study conducted at John Radcliffe Hospital, Oxford, UK)

## BEING BORN—AND WELCOMING YOUR BABY
*American Journal of Psychiatry*, "Childhood Traumas: An Outline and Overview", vol. 148, pp. 10–20

Bohus, Bela et al., "Oxytocin, Vasopressin and Memory: Opposite Effects on Consolidation and Retrieval Processes; Brain Research", vol. 157, pp. 414–417 (1978)

Chamberlain, Dr. David B., *The International Journal of Pre- and Perinatal Psychology and Medicine*, "What Babies Are Teaching Us About Violence", vol. 10/2, pp. 57–74

Cheek, D. B., *American Journal of Clinical Hypnosis*, "Sequential Head and Shoulder Movements Appearing with Age Regression in Hypnosis at Birth", vol. 16/4, pp. 261–266

Frederickson, R., *Repressed Memories* (Simon & Schuster, New York, 1992)

Grof, Stanislav, *The Realms of the Human Unconscious* (Souvenir Press, 1975)

Janov, Arthur, *The Feeling Child* (Sphere Books, 1977)

Janov, Arthur, *Imprints, the Lifelong Effects of the Birth Experience* (Coward-Cann Inc., New York, 1983)

Verny, Thomas, with Kelly, John, *The Secret Life of the Unborn Child* (Summit Books, 1981; Sphere Books, 1982; reprinted Warner Books, 1993)

Verny, Thomas, *The International Journal of Pre- and Perinatal Psychology and Medicine*, "Working with Pre- and Perinatal Material in Psychotherapy", vol. 8/3, pp. 161–183

## CAESAREAN BIRTH
Clements, Sarah, *The Caesarean Experience* (Pandora Publishing, UK, 1991)

Dickie, M., *Cesarean Births—Different Doorways to Life* (master's thesis, Smith College School for Social Work, Northampton, MA, USA, 1988)

Emerson, Dr. William, *Aesthema*, "Primal Therapy with Infants", vol. 7, pp. 13–27 (1987)

English, Dr. Jane, *Different Doorways—Adventures of a Cesarean-born* (Mount Shasta, Earth Heart, CA, 1986)

Francome, Dr. C., Savage, Professor W., Churchill, H., and Lewinson, H., *Caesarean Birth in Britain: A Book for Health Professionals and Parents* (Middlesex University Press, 1993)

Janov, Dr. Arthur, *Journal of Psychomatic Research*, "Towards a New Consciousness", vol. 21, pp. 333–339 (1977)

McCracken, Dennis, *Cesarean Personality Traits* (doctoral dissertation, Professional School of Psychology, San Francisco, CA, 1989)

Irving-Neto, Robyn L. and Verny, Thomas R., *The International Journal of Pre- and Perinatal Psychology and Medicine*, "Pre- and Perinatal Experiences and Personality: a Retrospective Analysis", pp. 139–172 (1992)

Verny, Thomas, *The International Journal of Pre- and Perinatal Psychology and Medicine*, "The Scientific Basis of Pre- and Perinatal Psychology", vol. 3, pp. 157–170

## YOUR AMAZING NEWBORN BABY
Appleton et al., *Review of Child Development Research*, "The Development of Behavioral Competence in Infancy", vol. 4 (Horowitz, F. D., ed., Chicago University Press, 1975)

Brazelton, T. B., *Seminars in Perinatology*, "Behavioral Competence in the Newborn Infant", vol. 3.3 (1979)

Brazelton, T. B., *Parent-Infant Relationships*, "Behavioral Competence in the Newborn Infant" (Taylor, P. M., ed., Grune & Stratton, New York, 1980)

DeCasper, A. and Fifer, W., *Science*, "Of Human Bonding: Newborns Prefer Their Mothers' Voices", vol. 208, pp. 1174–1176 (1980)

Illingworth, Ronald, *The Development of the Infant and Young Child*, "Abilities and Reflexes of the Newborn" chapter (Churchill Livingstone, Edinburgh, 1987)

Johnstone, Peter G. B., *The Newborn Child* (Churchill Livingstone, Edinburgh, 7th ed., 1994)

Lozoff et al., *Journal of Pediatrics*, "The Mother/Newborn Relationship; Limits of Adaptability", vol. 91, p. 1 (1977)

*Nature*, "Recognition of Mother's Voice in Early Infancy", vol. 79, p. 394 (1974)

*New Scientist*, "Mother's Face and the Newborn", vol. 61, p. 742 (1974)

Righard, L. and Alede, M., *Delivery Self Attachment* (video, 10 min., Geddes Productions, Sunland, California)

Truby, Henry, *Child Language*, "Prenatal and Neonatal Speech, Pre-speech and Infantile Speech Lexicon" (1975, special ed. of *Word* 27, parts 1–3)

\* *The Pre- and Perinatal Psychology Journal* has been renamed *The International Journal of Pre- and Perinatal Psychology and Medicine*. For ease, all other references give the new title.

# Glossary

**Alphafoetoprotein (AFP)**, protein circulating in the unborn baby's bloodstream, some of which crosses into the mother's bloodstream. By taking an ordinary blood sample from the mother it is possible to screen for the possibility of neural tube defects, such as spina bifida, as well as for Down's syndrome and some other chromosomal abnormalities.

**Amniocentesis**, safe, common, accurate, but invasive prenatal test, carried out between 11 and 18 weeks, to detect genetic abnormalities in the foetus, such as Down's syndrome. It involves painlessly taking a small sample of amniotic fluid, for analysis in the laboratory.

**Amniotic Fluid**, also known as "the waters", the clear liquid that surrounds your developing unborn baby when he or she is enclosed within the amniotic sac. The fluid cushions and protects the baby throughout pregnancy.

**Amniotic Sac**, the clear membrane sac which contains both the amniotic fluid and your developing baby.

**Apgar Score**, the 0- to 10-point scoring system for assessing your baby's well-being at birth.

**Birth Canal**, the unified passage formed by the uterus, the open/dilated cervix and the vagina, down which a baby passes as it is born. This open canal only exists during the second, or pushing, stage of labour, after which the cervix closes up again.

**Blastocyst**, a cell from one of the small group which has developed from the fusion of sperm and egg within three days of fertilization.

**Blastosphere** or **Blastula**, hollow, fluid-filled sphere made of blastocyst cells. It is this which implants itself in the lining of the womb (endometrium) to produce a pregnancy.

**Braxton Hicks Contractions**, gentle contractions that occur throughout pregnancy, as if your womb were limbering up and practising for labour.

**Caesarean Section** or **C-Section**, common, safe, but still major surgical operation whereby your baby is delivered via an incision in your abdominal and womb walls. It is usually carried out with an epidural anaesthetic so you can be awake to see your baby lifted out, but in emergencies it will be done under a general anaesthetic.

**Cervix**, the neck of the womb. When you are not pregnant it is almost closed, with a small canal called the Os through the middle measuring 1 to 2 mm across to allow menstrual flow to escape. Once pregnancy begins, it keeps the baby safely inside your womb. During childbirth it dilates to 10cm (4 inches) to allow the baby through.

**Chorionic Villus Sampling (CVS)**, alternative test for amniocentesis, the main advantage of which is that it can be done slightly earlier to check for certain genetic abnormalities.

**Chromosome**, tiny, threadlike, sausage-shaped structures made from a double strand of DNA coiled into a helix shape. Chromosomes are present in every cell of the body. Their job is to carry and transmit the cell's genetic information (which is a microcosm of the body to which it belongs) in the form of many thousands of separate genes.

**Colostrum**, the clear, nourishing pre-milk made by the breasts of pregnant, and newly delivered, mothers.

**Contraction**, the tightening and flexing of the womb's muscles during labour, which become more powerful (and usually more painful) as the childbirth progresses.

**Cordocentesis**, procedure involving taking a blood sample from the foetus through the wall of the mother's abdomen and womb, guided by ultrasound imaging. Cordocentesis (also called Umbilical Cord Sampling) is not done often, but is usually used to confirm abnormal or unusual findings from a CVS or amniocentesis test.

**Deoxyribonucleic Acid**, or **DNA**, the substance of which chromosomes are made.

**Doppler Ultrasound**, a technique used in ultrasound imaging to check on the development and behaviour of something which is moving, such as a beating embryonic heart, or foetal circulation.

**Ectopic Pregnancy**, also called a tubal pregnancy, problematic pregnancy that occurs when a blastosphere or early embryo implants itself in the wall of one of the Fallopian tubes leading from the ovary to womb, instead of its proper place in the lining of the womb itself.

**Embryo**, the future baby in its very earliest stages of development. Technically, just two cells which have resulted from a newly fertilized egg can be called an embryo. When it reaches the eight-week stage, it graduates to being called a foetus by doctors until it is born, when he or she will finally be referred to as a baby.

**Embryonic Disc**, the thickened, double-layered, biological sandwich which the embryo briefly develops into by day 11. This disc becomes a triple-layered living sandwich by day 14. Broadly speaking, the first layer becomes the skin, hair, ears and nervous system; the second develops into the intestine, respiratory system, liver and pancreas; and the third layer becomes body components such as the bones, muscles and circulatory system.

**Endometrium**, clinical term used to refer to the lining of the womb.

**Episiotomy**, a clean cut made under local anaesthetic in the perineum (the thickened muscular area between the anus and vaginal opening). It is carried out during a contraction, and is done to make more room for the baby's head to come out of the birth canal entrance.

**Foetus**, a prenate (unborn baby), between the 8 to 40 weeks developmental stages.

**Folic Acid**, member of the B-vitamin group, important for the workings of the central nervous system, and of vital importance to the unborn child—there is a significant link between shortage of folic acid in the mother and the chances of her having a baby with spina bifida.

**Fundus**, the upper part of the womb.

**Gene**, the biological unit of genetic inheritance, made from the nucleic acid DNA (see Deoxyribonucleic Acid).

**Human Chorionic Gonadotrophin (HCG)**, hormone which the chorionic villi (pre-placenta) make. HCG encourages your ovaries to produce extra oestrogen and progesterone to prepare the womb lining to receive your future baby and cuts down the reactivity of white blood cells, whose job it usually is to attack foreign matter in the body (there is always a danger that your body's defence cells may attack an early embryo because it is partially made up of foreign matter, i.e. your partner's). Thus HCG helps ensure your early embryo can implant safely in your womb lining.

*In Utero*, medical shorthand phrase often used in describing pregnancy and explaining embryology—it is Latin for "inside the womb".

**In Vitro Fertilization (IVF)**, the "Test Tube Baby" technique. IVF is a relatively high-tech method of helping couples who are experiencing considerable fertility difficulties in having a baby. It involves using drugs to stimulate the woman's ovaries to produce several ripe eggs, collecting those eggs under local anaesthetic, and placing them with a sample of her partner's sperm under laboratory conditions—usually in a sterile glass dish—so the sperm can fertilize the eggs. When they have done so, and the resulting early embryo has divided to reach the four- to eight-cell stage, these are carefully replaced inside the woman's womb, with the hope that they will implant and develop into one, two or even three foetuses. IVF often results in multiple births.

**Labour**, the process of childbirth.

**Lanugo**, the fine downy hair which appears, temporarily, on the baby's skin while he or she is inside the womb. It has usually disappeared by the time the baby is born, or will do so very soon afterwards.

**Lightening**, the welcome sensation many women report when their unborn baby settles down deeper into their pelvis, leaving more space in their upper abdomen. This makes breathing, which had become rather restricted as the lungs were being squashed by the baby's growing body, much easier for several weeks. It usually happens around weeks 34 to 36.

**Linea Nigra**, the fine line of darkened skin which appears around the 24th week of pregnancy, and extends from the top centre of the pubic hairline across the navel, and often reaches as far as the lower breastbone. It disappears soon after the baby is born.

**Neonatal**, the time span covering the first 28 days after birth.

**Neonate**, a baby from birth to 28 days of age.

**Oestrogen**, one of the female sex hormones, the levels of which rise dramatically during pregnancy.

**Ovary**, one of the pair of female gonads (glands producing reproductive cells). The ovaries are tucked deep inside the lower abdomen, beside the womb, to which they are each joined by a slim Fallopian tube.

**Ovulation**, the point when one of the ovaries releases a ripe egg. There is usually only one egg, though occasionally there may be two— as is the case with fraternal twins, where two separate sperm have fertilized two separate eggs.

**Perinatal**, literally, the "time around birth", a term used to describe anything to do with the time of giving birth/being born. In practice, it tends to be used to encompass the time from about the 24th week of pregnancy until a week after birth.

**Perineum**, the muscular area between the opening of the vagina and the rectum. It stretches considerably in front of the baby's head during the birth.

**Placenta**, the organ, grown by the embryo/foetus itself, which acts as a physical intermediary between the mother and her unborn baby's body. Food and oxygen travel across it in the bloodstream from mother to baby; waste products come back the other way, to be dealt with by the mother's kidneys and liver.

**Pre-eclampsia**, continuous raised blood pressure during pregnancy. This condition can adversely affect the growth of the unborn baby and can mean that it does not grow well and is born small (because it has not had quite enough food and oxygen *in utero*).

**Prenatal Psychology**, the psychology of unborn babies—the study of the development of their awareness, feelings and mental capabilities.

**Prenatal Sentience**, specifically, the awareness ("sentient" meaning intelligent or knowing) of unborn babies.

**Prenate** or **Preborn**, blanket terms often used as alternatives to "foetus", "embryo" or "unborn baby", meaning the unborn child at any stage of development.

**Progesterone**, sex hormone vital to the maintenance of any pregnancy.

**Quickening**, traditional word for the point when the mother first begins to feel her baby move inside her.

**Rebirthing**, psychotherapeutic technique in which a person is helped to remember and re-experience the emotions and circumstances of his or her own birth. Rebirthing can involve light hypnosis, breathing techniques, guided imagery and deep relaxation and symbolic physical re-enactment.

**Startle (Moro) Reflex**, one of the important early reflexes babies have at birth.

**Stretch Marks**, fine red lines which can appear quite suddenly on the skin covering any rapidly expanding areas during pregnancy, such as the abdomen, breasts and sometimes the upper thighs (skin being pulled from the abdomen area). Doctors call them stria and they are in fact scar tissue. They fade to silvery marks within a few months of delivery.

**Trophoblast**, the outer wall of the blastocyst (see above), which produces tiny seeking fronds called villi. Its job is to help the early embryo implant itself into the lining of the womb, and to supply it with food. The villi from the trophoblast proliferate rapidly and develop into the placenta.

**Ultrasound**, method of looking at the foetus using sound waves. Sensitive ultrasound equipment, particularly if used intravaginally, can also detect an embryo from four or five weeks of age while it is in the womb.

**Umbilical Cord**, the unborn baby's lifeline. It connects him or her, via the umbilicus, to the placenta. The cord contains two arteries and one vein which bring food and oxygen in, as well as taking waste products out to be dealt with by the mother's system.

**Umbilical Cord Sampling**, see **Cordocentesis**.

**Uterus**, the womb, the muscular little organ which contains the growing baby. It stretches from the size and shape of a very small pear to that of a king-sized watermelon, so that the baby can grow from a small bundle made up of a few cells into a separate person. The uterus also contains the placenta, amniotic sac and amniotic fluid. During labour it is the muscles of the uterus which contract powerfully to push the baby out.

**Vernix**, rich, greasy material which covers the baby's skin *in utero*.

**Womb**, see **Uterus**.

## PHOTOGRAPHIC ACKNOWLEDGEMENTS

**KEY: SPL/Science Photo Library**
Emap/Elan 76 top, 66, 95, 104, 130, 131 left, 141
Impact/Morton 11, /Penn 116,
Rex Features 5, 105, 129, 136, 145
Rex/SIPA 82, 124, 127, 132, 137, 144 top
Rex/Oler 73 bot, /Rastellini 133
SPL 45 top right
SPL/BSIP 17 top, 51 top, 64 right
SPL/Biophotos 9 right
SPL/Brain 10 top, 14 top
SPL/Burgess 75 left
SPL/CC Studio 28
SPL/CNR1 9 left, 43, 75 right

SPL/Custom Med
134SPL/Sutherland
SPL/Eward 8
SPL/Griem 148
SPL/Jerrican 146
SPL/Kjeldsen 18 top
SPL/Kulyk 53 bot, 84
SPL/Leca 139 both pictures
SPL/Leroy 6, 12/13
SPL/McIntyre 23
SPL/Meadows 81 left,114, 119
SPL/Motta 12, 15, 16, 18 bot, 19, 20, 21 inset, 34 top, 34 center, 44, 45 top left,45 bot 64 left
SPL/Nikas 21 main
SPL/Percival 7 bot, 135 both

pictures
SPL/Petit Format: 1, 7 top, 10 bot, 31, 33 bot, 34 b ot, 34/5, 36, 37 all pictures, 38, 39 all pictures, 40/41 all pictures, 56 top, 67, 68, 69 all pictures, 70 all pictures, 79 top right, 131 right/Henstra 144 bot
SPL/Rawlins 17 bot
SPL/Saada 50, 73 top, 78, 79, bot right
SPL/Salisbury Hosp 33 top, 107 top
SPL/Saturn Stills 51 bot, 52, 80
SPL/Schatten 14 bot
SPL/Tsiaras 30, 32
SPL/Walker 29 top, 29 bot
Zefa 22, 24 top, 26 top right, 27,

42, 55, 56 bot, 57, 72, 76, 81 right,82, 85, 91, 92,107 bot, 118, 130/1, 147, 148 top, 149, 150/1
Zefa/Benser 117
Zefa/Jonas 24
Zefa/Kotoh 26 bot
Zefa/Lenz 24 top inset
Zefa/Norman 94
Zefa/Pacific Stock 25 bot
Zefa/Rossi 53 top, 115, 125,
Zefa/Sander 94
Zefa/Stockmarket 7 right, 26 top left, 74, 76 bot, 79 left, 142/3

# Index